Bioactive Phytochemicals: Drug Discovery to Product Development

Edited by

Javed Ahmad

College of Pharmacy,
Najran University,
KSA

Co-editor

Javed Ahamad

Department of Pharmacognosy,
Faculty of Pharmacy,
Tishk International University,
Kurdistan Region, Erbil,
Iraq

Bioactive Phytochemicals: Drug Discovery to Product Development

Editor: Javed Ahmad

Co-editor: Javed Ahamad

ISBN (Online): 978-981-14-6448-5

ISBN (Print): 978-981-14-6446-1

ISBN (Paperback): 978-981-14-6447-8

Published by Bentham Science Publishers Pte. Ltd. Singapore. All Rights Reserved.

need for a court order if at any point you breach any terms of this License Agreement. In no event will any delay or failure by Bentham Science Publishers in enforcing your compliance with this License Agreement constitute a waiver of any of its rights.

3. You acknowledge that you have read this License Agreement, and agree to be bound by its terms and conditions. To the extent that any other terms and conditions presented on any website of Bentham Science Publishers conflict with, or are inconsistent with, the terms and conditions set out in this License Agreement, you acknowledge that the terms and conditions set out in this License Agreement shall prevail.

Bentham Science Publishers Pte. Ltd.
80 Robinson Road #02-00
Singapore 068898
Singapore
Email: subscriptions@benthamscience.net

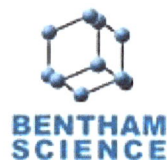

**BENTHAM
SCIENCE**

CONTENTS

FOREWORD

Plants have always considered been as 'Nature's Library' for new chemical entities and one of the major resources in drug discovery and new drug development. Medicinal plants that have been used in traditional systems of medicine are being studied more than a fine decade for scientific evaluation and validation of the application, which provides rational and evidence-based alternative medicines and eventually a backbone of modern day's herbal drug, herbal bioactives, semisynthetic and to some extent in synthetic drug and pharmaceutical industries.

In the light of the foregoing, this Book, "Bioactive Phytochemicals: Drug Discovery to Product Development" is a tremendously important and in-depth contribution to the subject of Phyto-pharmaceuticals from drug discovery to product development. The book has brought together diverse works in the scientific literature under an umbrella on the use of therapeutically active phytochemicals in the treatment of various chronic disorders. An excellent effort has been made in this frankly speaking 'a much-needed book' to address the challenges in plant and plant bioactive based drug development to its transition to the phytopharmaceutical product comprehensively and sequentially. I am confident that the book is capable of centering the attention of the reader on the limitless potentials of bioactive phytochemicals. It does particularly well too in highlighting several current areas of interest in extraction, isolation, structural characterization, pharmacological screening, product development and regulatory perspectives of herbal drugs and bioactive phytochemicals.

I have, no doubt, that this book will be well-received (equally) by the researchers in the phytopharmaceutical industry and academia. Moreover, this book is really good at offering a vast knowledge on this subject to the chemist and pharmacy students.

Dr. Sohail Akhter
Principal Scientist
New Product development, Global R & D
Teva Pharmaceuticals
Runcorn, United Kingdom

PREFACE

Early man explored natural surroundings such as plants, animals, and minerals to find the remedies of different ailments. An alternative system of medicines such as Ayurveda, Unani, Kampo, and traditional Chinese medicinal products are used as dietary supplements and nutraceuticals reported to become a major part in the treatment of chronic disorders such as diabetes, cancer, malaria, arthritis, inflammation, liver disorders, and cardiac disorders. WHO Traditional Medicine Programme is also designed on the potential of ethnomedicine as a lead for drug discovery. Compounds from plants have been extracted to investigate novel therapeutics since the origin of medicine. Natural bioactive compounds from medicinal plants are inexplicably diverse in chemical structure, biological properties and the unmet therapeutic requirements attribute to develop an interest in the reemergence of bioactive natural compounds that will lead to isolation, structural characterization and finding pharmaceutical activity.

The book discusses the scope and approaches of drug discovery from natural products; cultivation, collection and processing of medicinal plants; Methods and high throughput techniques for extraction, isolation, and characterization of bioactive phytochemicals; pharmacological screening for its activity and formulation development as well as quality control of natural medicinal products. It also discusses the regulations specified for natural medicinal products in a different region of the world. The last chapter of the book is devoted to discuss the role of natural herbal products for the treatment of human diseases such as cancer, cardiovascular diseases, diabetes, obesity, inflammation, and neurological disorders. Each chapter concludes with a general reference section, which is a bibliographic guide to more advanced texts.

This book will provide in-depth information and comprehensive discussion on extraction, isolation, structural characterization, pharmacological screening of bioactive phytochemicals as well as product development and regulatory perspective of herbal medicine. Researchers, industries, and students would be interested in this concise body of information. The contributing authors are drawn from a rich blend of experts in various areas of herbal medicine encompass drug discovery to product development.

Dr. Javed Ahmad
College of Pharmacy
Najran University
KSA

Co-editor

Javed Ahamad
Department of Pharmacognosy,
Faculty of Pharmacy,
Tishk International University,
Kurdistan Region, Erbil,
Iraq

List of Contributors

Abdul Samad — Department of Pharmaceutical Chemistry, Faculty of Pharmacy, Tishk International University, Kurdistan Region, Iraq

Afrin Salma — Department of Pharmaceutical Chemistry, Translum Institute of Pharmaceutical Education and Research, Meerut (UP), India

Ahmed Nawaz Khan — School of Pharmacy, Graphic Era Hill University, Dehradun Uttarakhand, 248002, India

Asad Ali — Department of Chemistry, School of Chemical and Life Sciences, Jamia Hamdard University, New Delhi, India

Chandra Kala — Faculty of Pharmacy, Maulana Azad University, Jodhpur, Rajasthan, 342802, India

Dinesh Kumar Patel — Department of Pharmaceutical Science, Sam Higginbottom, University of Agricultural Tech. and Science, India

Esra T. Anwer — Department of Pharmaceutics, Faculty of Pharmacy, Tishk International University, Kurdistan Region, Iraq

Faraat Ali — Laboratory Services, Botswana Medicines Regulatory Authority, Plot 112 International Finance Park, Gaborone, Botswana

Govind Prasad Dubey — Study Director and Coordinator - Collaborative Program, Institute of Medical Sciences, Banaras Hindu University, Varansi, India

Jamia Firdous — Department of Pharmacy, Institute of Bio-Medical Education and Research, Mangalayatan University, Aligarh, India

Jaswanth Albert — Faculty of Pharmacology, Surabhi Dayakar Rao College of Pharmacy, Gajwel, Rimmanaguda, Hyderabad, Telangana, India

Javed Ahamad — Department of Pharmacognosy, Faculty of Pharmacy, Tishk International University, Erbil, Kurdistan Region, Iraq

Javed Ahmad — Department of Pharmaceutics, College of Pharmacy, Najran University, Kingdom of Saudi Arabia

Kamna Sharma — Department of Pharmaceutical Analysis, Indo-Soviet Friendship College of Pharmacy, Moga, Punjab, India

Kamran Javed Naquvi — Department of Pharmacognosy & Phytochemistry, Faculty of Pharmaceutical Sciences, Rama University, Rama City, Mandhana, Kanpur (Uttar Pradesh) - 209 217, India

Manisha Trivedi — NIMS University, Jaipur, Rajasthan, India

Mohammad Shabib Akhtar — Department of Clinical Pharmacy, College of Pharmacy, Najran University, Najran, Kingdom of Saudi Arabia

Muath Sh. Mohammed Ameen — Department of Pharmaceutics, Faculty of Pharmacy, Tishk International University, Kurdistan Region, Iraq

Naila Hassan Ali Alkefai — Department of Pharmacognosy, Faculty of Pharmacy, University of Hafer Albatin, Hafer Albatin, KSA

Nehal Mohsin — Department of Clinical Pharmacy, College of Pharmacy, Najran University, Najran, Kingdom of Saudi Arabia

Omji Porwal Department of Pharmacognosy, Faculty of Pharmacy, Tishk International University, Erbil, Kurdistan Region, Iraq

Raad A Kaskoos Faculty of Pharmacy, Howler Medical University, Kurdistan Region, Iraq

Rahul Tripathi Medpharm Pharmaceutical Ltd., Guilford, United Kingdom

Sachin Singh School of pharmaceutical Sciences, Lovely professional University, Phagwara-144411, Punjab, India

Saurabh Gupta Department of Pharmacology, Chitkara University, Jansla, Rajpura, Punjab 140401, India

Shaik Khasimbi Department of Pharmaceutical Chemistry, Delhi Institute of Pharmaceutical Sciences and Research (DIPSAR), Mehrauli-Badarpur Road, PushVihar, Sector-3, New Delhi, 110017, India

Shankar Katekhaye Center for pharmaceutical Engineering Science University of Barford, Barford-BD71DP, United Kingdom

Shehla Nasar Mir Najibullah Department of Pharmacognosy, Faculty of Pharmacy, King Khalid University, Abha, KSA

Showkat R. Mir Department of Pharmacognosy, School of Pharmaceutical Education and Research, Jamia Hamdard, New Delhi, India

Subasini Uthirapathy Department of Pharmacology, Faculty of Pharmacy, Tishk International University, KRG, Iraq

Tara Fuad Tahir Faculty of Science and Health, Koya University, Kurdistan Region, Iraq

CHAPTER 1

Drug Discovery from Plant Sources: Scope, Approach and Challenges

Javed Ahmad[1] and **Javed Ahamad**[2,*]

[1] *Department of Pharmaceutics, College of Pharmacy, Najran University, Kingdom of Saudi Arabia*

[2] *Department of Pharmacognosy, Faculty of Pharmacy, Tishk International University, Erbil, Kurdistan Region, Iraq*

Abstract: Medicinal plants are recognized to fulfill human necessities like food, clothes, shelter and health. The search for eternal health and longevity to seek remedy to relieve discomfort prompted mankind to develop many ways and means of health care systems. Traditional medicines were practiced in ancient civilizations for the cure of ailments. In recent years, natural products play a very important role in drug discovery for life-threatening ailments like cancer, malaria, diabetes and cardiovascular problems. Recently, drug discovery from plants for the treatment of cancer gets more focused and leads to the discovery of novel anticancer drugs such as paclitaxel, docetaxel, topotecan, irinotecan, vincristine and vinblastine. Drug discovery from plants is a long and tedious process, and it requires selecting suitable plants, pre-clinical screening, clinical evaluation and drug approval for marketing. Herbal medicines obtained from plants are generally considered safe compared to synthetic drugs, and secondary metabolites obtained from plants have more chemical diversity and considered superior to synthetic combinatorial chemicals. In this book chapter, we comprehensively discussed the advantages and role of higher plants in drug discovery, steps and approaches of drug discovery from higher plants.

Keywords: Approaches of Drug Discovery, Cancer, Drug Discovery, Diabetes, Malaria, Natural Products, Plants.

1. INTRODUCTION

Since ancient times, plants are recognized to fulfill human necessities like food, clothes, shelter and remedies for ailments. Since the early days, mankind explored natural resources and used them as a remedy for the cure of diseases. The traditional systems of medicine such as Ayurveda, Unani, Chinese medicine and

* **Corresponding author Dr. Javed Ahamad:** Department of Pharmacognosy, Faculty of Pharmacy, Tishk International University, Erbil, Kurdistan Region, Iraq; E-mails: jas.hamdard@gmail.com, javed.ahamad@tiu.edu.iq

Homeopathy are examples of ways of treatment of human diseases. In ancient times, the human beings used natural resources for various purposes, such as food and medicinal agents [1]. Traditional medicines were practiced in ancient civilizations; the traditional practitioner gathered knowledge from generation to generation, and sometimes they document this knowledge. Ancient Indian scholars such as Charaka and Sushrutha, examined and classified medicinal herbs based on their properties and they called it as "Gunas". Charaka arranged 50 groups containing ten herbs in each group, and according to him, these herbs are sufficient to cure all types of human diseases. Sushrutha also prepared seven groups from 760 herbs based upon some common properties [2]. Chinese scholars also worked meticulously and developed remedies from natural resources. One of the oldest known literature by *Pent Sao* documented by ShenNung around 3000 B.C., and it contained 365 drugs, one for each day of the year [3]. Hippocrates *"Father of medicine"* (460-360 B.C.), Aristotle (384-322 B.C.), Dioscorides (40-80 A.D.), Galen (131-200 A.D.) and the early Arabian physicians like Rhazes (865-925 AD) and Avicenna (980-1037 AD) were recognized as pioneers in drug discovery from natural products [4].

Higher plants have advantages in drug discovery compared to synthetic drugs because they have a long history of use by humans as food and spices. Natural products obtained from plants are generally considered safe compared to synthetic drugs, and the secondary metabolites obtained from plants have more chemical diversity and considered superior to synthetic combinatorial chemicals [5]. Several natural products recently showed cytotoxic and antitumor activities in clinical trials and were successfully developed as anticancer drugs such as vincristine, vinblastine, paclitaxel and docetaxeletc. Drug discovery from plants today is an expensive and lengthy process. The drug discovery from plants requires a team effort consisting of experts from different disciplines such as pharmacognosists, pharmacologists, medicinal chemist and pharmaceutics. Phytochemicals from medicinal plants serve as a lead compound in drug discovery and are further used for synthetic or semi-synthetic drug development to ensure patent protection [6]. In ancient civilization, plants were used as medicinal agents for the treatment of various human ailments. The knowledge of medicinal values of these plants was inherited from generation to generation. Most of these traditional practitioners formulate and dispense their own medicines; hence this requires proper documentation and research to use natural products as therapeutically effective and safe medicinal agents [7]. In recent years, traditional medicines have emerged as an alternative treatment of chronic diseases and lifestyle disorders such as cancer, malaria, tuberculosis, diabetes, obesity and cardiovascular complications [8]. Drug discovery from the plant is a long and tedious process, and it requires selecting suitable plants, biological or pre-clinical screening, clinical evaluation and drug approval for marketing. In this book chapter, we comprehensively discussed the advantages and role of higher plants in drug discovery, steps and approaches of drug discovery from higher plants.

2. ADVANTAGES OF DRUG DISCOVERY FROM NATURAL RESOURCES

Newman and Cragg, reported that totally 1562 new drugs approved during 1981 to 2014, of which, those of plant origin comprised as follows: natural products (4%; N), derivatives of natural products (21%, ND), synthetic compounds with natural product-derived pharmacophores (10%; S*/NM), and synthetic drug with NP pharmacophore (11%; S/NM). It is clear from the above report that natural products contribute a lot in drug discovery [9]. Plants are considered as equal or superior in drug discovery because of their chemical diversity and human friendly in nature based on their long history of use as food by a human. Phytochemicals have been elaborated within living systems, they are often perceived as showing more drug-likeness and biological friendliness or tolerance than synthetic molecules, making bioactive phytochemicals good candidates for further drug discovery and development [6]. The data on new drugs approved during 1981-2014 is summarized in Table **1** and Fig. (**1**).

Table 1. New drugs approved during 1981-2014 from all sources (number = 1562).

Code	Category	Numbers	Percentage
B	Biological drugs	250	16%
N	Natural drugs	67	4%
NB	Botanical drugs with defined mixture	9	1%
ND	Natural product derivatives	320	21%
S	Synthetic drugs	420	27%
S/NM	Synthetic drug with NP pharmacophore	172	11%
S*	Synthetic drugs which mimics natural product	61	4%
S*/NM	Synthetic compounds with natural product-derived pharmacophores	162	10%
V	Vaccine	101	6%
T	Total	1562	100%

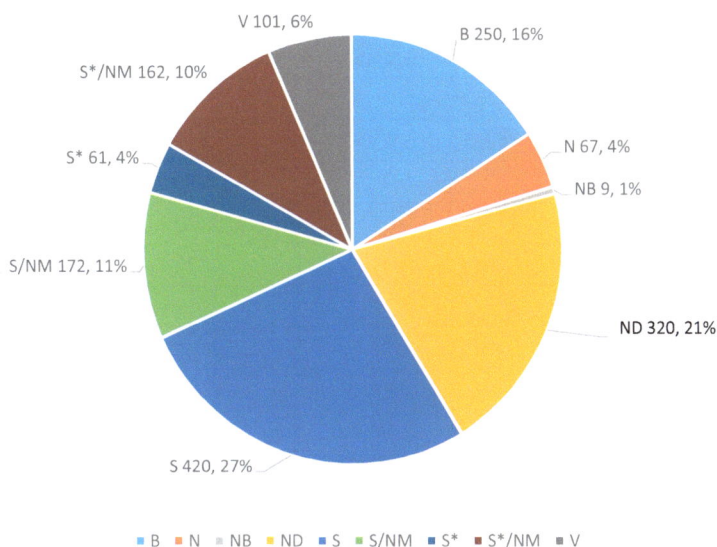

Fig. (1). New drugs approved during 1981-2014 from all sources (number = 1562) [9].

3. ROLE OF MEDICINAL PLANTS IN DRUG DISCOVERY

Higher medicinal plants considered a good candidate in drug discovery because of long use as food. A rough estimate of about 65% world population relies on traditional medicines for their primary health care needs. Newman *et al.*, reported that drug discovered from the natural product or natural product derivatives comprises about 26% of all new chemical entities launched into the market between 1981 to 2014 [9]. WHO-Traditional Medicine Programme is based on the potential of ethnomedicine as a lead for drug discovery [10]. Farnsworth *et al.*, conducted a survey worldwide and identified 122 phytocompounds from traditionally used plants, and he found that about 80% of these phytochemicals were used for the same or related ethnomedical purposes. The authors also found that these phytochemicals were derived only from 94 species of medicinal plants [1, 5]. Up to 122 phytochemicals are derived only from 94 species of plants, whereas there is an abundant number of plant species not explored phytochemically and pharmacologically [1]. Several workers estimated the number of plants on the planet, which is about 250,000, and out of these, only about 6% have been screened for biologic activity and 15% have been evaluated phytochemically, so there is an abundance of drugs remaining to be discovered in these plants [11]. Some important natural drugs/phytochemicals, which are derived from higher plants, are summarized in Table **2**.

Table 2. Bioactive phytochemicals derived from higher plants [1, 5].

S. No.	Plant source	Phytochemicals	Pharmacological or clinical use
1.	*Adonis vernalis* L.	Adoniside	Cardiotonic
2.	*Aesculus hippocastanum* L.	Aescin	Anti-inflammatory
3.	*Agrimonia eupatoria* L.	Agrimophol	Anthelmintic
4.	*Ammi majus* L.	Xanthotoxin	Leukoderma; vitiligo
5.	*Ammi visnaga* L.	Khellin	Bronchodilator
6.	*Anamirtacocculus* L.	Picrotoxin	Analeptic
7.	*Ananascomosus* L.	Bromelain	Anti-inflammatory
8.	*Andrographis paniculata* Nees	Andrographolide	Bacillary dysentery
9.	*Anisodus tanguticus* Maxim.	Anisodamine, Anisodine	Anticholinergic
10.	*Ardisia japonica* Bl.	Bergenin	Antitussive
11.	*Areca catechu* L.	Arecoline	Anthelmintic
12.	*Artemisia maritima* L.	Santonin	Ascaricide
13.	*Artemisia annua* L.	Artemisinin	Antimalarial
14.	*Atropa belladonna* L.	Atropine	Anticholinergic
15.	*Berberis vulgaris* L.	Berberine	Bacillary dysentery
16.	*Brassica nigra* L.	Allyl isothiocyanate	Rubefacient
17.	*Camptotheca acuminata* D	Camptothecin	Anticancer
18.	*Camellia sinensis* L.	Caffeine Theophylline	CNS stimulant Diuretic; bronchodilator
19.	*Carica papaya* L.	Papain, Chymopapain	Proteolytic; mucolytic
20.	*Catharanthus roseus* L.	Vincristine, Vinblastine	Anticancer
21.	*Cassia spp.*	Sennosides A & B	Laxative
22.	*Centella asiatica* L.	Asiaticoside	Vulnerary, nervine tonic
23.	*Cephaelis ipecacuanha*	Emetine	Amoebicide; emetic
24.	*Chondodendron tomentosum*	Tubocurarine	Skeletal muscle relaxant
25.	*Cinchona spp.*	Quinine Quinidine	Antimalarial Antiarrhythmic
26.	*Colchicum autumnale* L.	Colchicine	Antitumor agent; antigout
27.	*Convallaria majalis* L.	Convallotoxin	Cardiotonic
28.	*Crotolaria sessiliflora* L.	Monocrotaline	Antitumor agent
29.	*Curcuma longa* L.	Curcumin	Choleretic
30.	*Cynara scolymus* L.	Cynarin	Choleretic
31.	*Datura metel* L.	Scopolamine	Sedative

S. No.	Plant source	Phytochemicals	Pharmacological or clinical use
32.	*Digenea simplex* Wulf.	Kainic Acid	Ascaricide
33.	*Digitalis lanata* Ehrh.	Lanatosides A, B, C Acetyldigoxin, Deslanoside, Digoxin	Cardiotonic
34.	*Digitalis purpurea* L.	Digoxin, Digitoxin, Gitalin	Cardiotonic
35.	*Ephedra sinica* Stapf.	Ephedrine, Pseudoephedrine	Sympathomimetic
36.	*Erythroxylum coca* Lamk.	Cocaine	Local anaesthetic
37.	*Fraxinus rhynchophylla* Hance	Aesculetin	Antidysentery
38.	*Glycyrrhiza glabra* L.	Glycyrrhizin	Sweetener
39.	*Gossypium spp.*	Gossypol	Male contraceptive
40.	*Hydrangea macrophylla*	Phyllodulcin	Sweetener
41.	*Hydrastis canadensis* L.	Hydrastine	Hemostatic; astringent
42.	*Hyoscamus niger* L.	Hyoscamine	Anticholinergic
43.	*Lobelia inflata* L.	Lobeline	Smoking deterrent; respiratory stimulant
44.	*Papaver somniferum* L.	Morphine; Codeine, Noscapine	Analgesic; Antitussive
45.	*Pausinystalia yohimbe*	Yohimbine	Aphrodisiac
46.	*Physostigma venenosum* Balf.	Physostigmine	Cholinesterase inhibitor
47.	*Pilocarpus jaborandi* Holmes	Pilocarpine	Parasympathomimetic
48.	*Podophyllum peltatum* L.	Etoposide, Teniposide Podophyllotoxin	Antitumor agent
49.	*Potentilla fragaroides* L.	(+)-Catechin	Haemostatic
50.	*Rauvolfia serpentina* L.	Ajmalicine	Circulatory disorders
51.	*Rauvolfia serpentina* L.	Reserpine	Antihypertensive; tranqulizer
52.	*Salix alba* L.	Salicin	Analgesic
53.	*Silybum marianum* L.	Silymarin	Antihepatotoxic
54.	*Simarouba glauca* DC.	Glaucaroubin	Amoebicide
55.	*Stephania sinica* Diels	Rotundine	Analgesic; sedative
56.	*Stevia rebaudiana*	Stevioside	Sweetener
57.	*Strophanthus gratus* Baill.	Ouabain	Cardiotonic
58.	*Strychnos nux-vomica* L.	Strychnine	CNS stimulant
59.	*Taxus brevifolia* Nutt.	Taxol	Anticancer
60.	*Theobroma cacao* L.	Theobromine	Diuretic; bronchodilator
61.	*Thymus vulgaris* L.	Trichosanthin	Abortifacient
62.	*Urginea maritima* L.	Scillarin A	Cardiotonic

(Table 2) cont.....

S. No.	Plant source	Phytochemicals	Pharmacological or clinical use
63.	*Valeriana officinalis* L.	Valepotriates	Sedative
64.	*Veratrum album* L.	Protoveratrines A & B	Antihypertensive

4. STEPS OF DRUG DISCOVERY FROM HIGHER PLANTS

Drug discovery and development from plants require multidisciplinary research that includes experts from the natural product, pharmacology and pharmaceutics. For drug discovery from higher medicinal plants, the following three important steps are required: (a) selection of appropriate plant candidates for biological evaluation; (b) development of specific methods for biological evaluations (pre-clinical and clinical models); and bioassay-guided fractionation and isolation of new bioactive phytocompounds and their structure elucidation.

The drug discovery and development takes a long time and is expensive. According to Shrager, drug discovery involves several steps. The first step is to find a 'lead' molecule. Lead from plants is a bioactive molecule, which exhibits desired biological or pharmacological activity and safety in cytotoxicity tests in the suitable *in-vitro* model [12]. The discovery of lead molecules from higher plants includes the screening of large numbers of plants pharmacologically and then fractionation and isolation of particular phytochemicals. This isolated new molecule with desired pharmacological activity serves as a lead molecule in drug discovery. In the next step, animal safety analysis is done to determine whether the lead compound is toxic (toxicity test), and then the *in-vivo* effectiveness of the lead molecule against disease in an animal model was evaluated (Fig. **2**). The pre-clinical studies usually done in animal models and clinical studies in human subjects. If these pre-clinical and clinical tests give positive results, then the next step is to design proper dosage forms. In the last step of drug development, the new drug is applied for a license to get marketing rights [6].

5. DRUG DISCOVERY FROM HIGHER PLANTS: APPROACHES

Higher plants have immense medicinal values, and they should be pharmacologically evaluated for the treatment of complicated diseases like cancer, HIV/AIDS, CVD, diabetes, *etc*. Successful strategies for selecting plant candidate for isolation, characterization and drug discovery involves the selection of plants based upon ethnomedicinal use. There are four main approaches usually used to select proper medicinal plants in drug discovery and development [1, 6, 13].

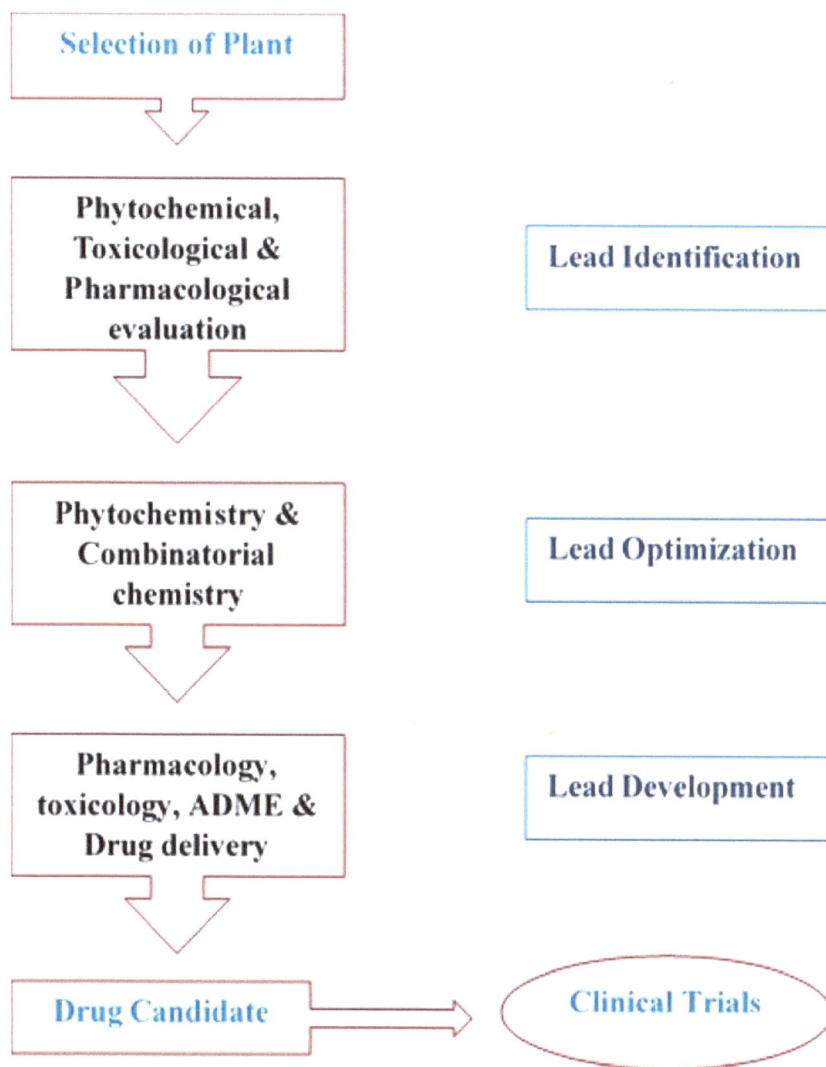

Fig. (2). Drug discovery from medicinal plants.

5.1. Ethno-Pharmacological Approach

Ethnomedicine may be defined as the "use of medicinal plants by human". Since ancient times, humans preserved natural resources, which they used as a remedy for the cure of diseases. This traditional knowledge now became a very important criterion for the selection of plants in drug discovery. In this approach of drug discovery, a diversified means are applied, such as observation, description and experimental evaluation of indigenous plants. It also includes the role of ethnobotany, phytochemistry, and pharmacology that contribute to drug discovery [1, 5]. Farnsworth *et al.*, identified 122 phytocompounds used worldwide are derived from traditionally used plants. He also suggested the following steps of drug discovery from traditional plants based upon their ethnopharmacological use (Fig. 3) [5].

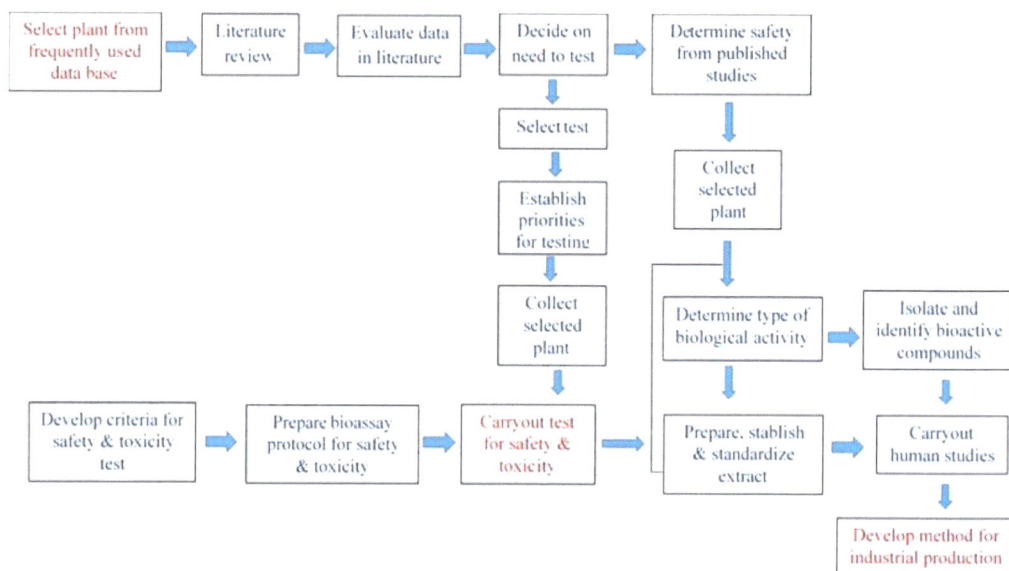

Fig. (3). Flow chart of drug discovery based upon ethno-pharmacology.

5.2. Follow-up of Pharmacological Reports

Pharmacological or biological activities are reported in the literature from the 1930s to 1970s and contain pharmacological data, and unfortunately, they were not screened or evaluated phytochemically. A rough estimate of a number of plants on the planet is about 250,000, and out of these, only about 6% have been screened for pharmacologic activity and 15% have been evaluated phytochemically, so there is an abundance of drugs yet to be discovered in these plants [11]. These literature reports are a very good basis for the selection of a plant candidate in drug discovery and the development of a new drug.

5.3. Random Selection Followed by Phytochemical Screening

This method of drug discovery, also called as phytochemical screening approach, it has been used in the past and is currently pursued mainly in the developing countries for initial stages of drug discovery for selection of the particular class of plant species based upon their secondary metabolites [1]. These phytochemical tests are simple to perform, but sometimes the accuracy of these phytochemicals tests is not reliable, and it makes it difficult to assess the correct idea about the pharmacological activity of medicinal plants [14].

5.4. Random Selection Followed by Pharmacological Screening

In this method of drug discovery, medicinal plants were selected randomly and evaluated against several diseases. This method reduces the bias in collecting plant samples based on ethnomedical data. In this approach, plant samples are submitted to routine extraction, isolation, and systemic pharmacological assay without a preconceived selection on the basis of ethnobotanical knowledge [5]. The National Cancer Institute (NCI) in the United States and Central Drug Research Institute (CDRI) in India are examples of such sponsored programs for the discovery of drugs from natural products. NCI screened about 35,000 species of medicinal plants from 1960 to 1981; this extensive research resulted in the discovery of two potent anticancer drugs: taxol and camptothecin [15]. In India, at CDRI, about 2,000 plants were screened pharmacologically for various biological activities, till date, no active biological molecule was identified from this research [16]. The disadvantage of this approach is the very low probability of finding a lead compound per plant species investigated.

6. CHALLENGES IN DRUG DISCOVERY FROM HIGHER PLANTS

The drug discovery and development from natural resources poses significant challenges in several areas. The first most important concern is the supply of the drug in sufficient quantities to allow pre-clinical and clinical evaluations and, ultimately, if the given drug is a success in clinical outcomes, then commercial production. The second major challenge is that of formulation, as natural products from plant origin are mostly insoluble in an aqueous phase, and such solubility is an important requirement for the administration of the drug to humans [17].

There are several other disadvantages of using plants in drug discovery, such as plants as biologic systems have inherent potential variability in their chemistry and resulting in pharmacological activity [18]. Since 1992, several countries prohibited the collection and export of indigenous plant materials. It was also reported that in areas where regulations permit plant collection and export, at least 2 years are required to negotiate and obtain permission to collect plant materials. Several other restrictions for drug discovery from natural resources include: (a) intellectual property rights, (b) preservation of genetic materials, and (c) compensation for drug discoveries arising from natural resources. The authors also reported that drug discovery from natural resources is time-consuming and costly [19]. The drug discovery and development of new drugs cost approximately 2.6 billion USD [20].

CONCLUDING REMARKS

Higher plants are considered equal or superior in drug discovery because of their chemical diversity and human-friendly nature based on their long history of use as food by a human. Phytochemicals have been elaborated within living systems; they are often perceived as showing more drug-likeness and biological friendliness than synthetic molecules, making bioactive phytochemicals good candidates for further drug discovery and development. Medicinal plants are considered as a novel source of phytochemicals, which are equal or superior in drug discovery and development program, *e.g.*, artemisinin, vinblastine, vincristine, camptothecin, quinine, morphine, taxol, and digoxin. Natural products played a very important role in drug discovery and development, as a total of 1562 new drugs approved from 1981 to 2014, out of which natural products and natural product derivatives were about 51%. Due to recent advances in the field of extraction, isolation, characterization and pharmacological screening methods, drug discovery from natural products become very fast. In recent decades, more and more drugs were discovered from natural products.

ABBREVIATIONS

B = Biological drugs
CDRI = Central Drug Research Institute
N = Natural drugs
NB = Botanical drugs with defined mixture
ND = Natural product derivatives
NCI = National Cancer Institute
S = Synthetic drugs
S/NM = Synthetic drug with NP pharmacophore
S* = Synthetic drugs which mimic of natural product
S*/NM = Synthetic compounds with natural product-derived pharmacophores
V = Vaccine
WHO = World health organization

CONSENT FOR PUBLICATION

Not applicable.

CONFLICT OF INTEREST

The authors confirm that this chapter content has no conflict of interest.

ACKNOWLEDGEMENTS

Declared none.

REFERENCES

[1]   Fabricant DS, Farnsworth NR. The value of plants used in traditional medicine for drug discovery. Environ Health Perspect 2001; 109 (Suppl. 1): 69-75.
[PMID: 11250806]

[2]   Patwardhan B, Vaidya ADB, Chorghade M. Ayurveda and natural products drug discovery. Curr Sci 2004; 86(6): 789-99.

[3]   Bannerman RHO, Burton J, Ch'en WC. Traditional Medicine and Health Care Coverage: A Reader for Health Administrators and Practitioners. Geneva: World Health Organization 1983.

[4]   Trease and Evans, Pharmacognosy. 16th ed., Evans WC. Saunders Publication London: Elsevier 2009.

[5]   Farnsworth NR, Akerele O, Bingel AS, Soejarto DD, Guo Z. Medicinal plants in therapy. Bull World Health Organ 1985; 63(6): 965-81.
[PMID: 3879679]

[6]   Lahlou M. Screening of natural products for drug discovery. Expert Opin Drug Discov 2007; 2(5): 697-705.
[http://dx.doi.org/10.1517/17460441.2.5.697] [PMID: 23488959]

[7]   Dubey NK, Kumar R, Tripathi P. Global promotion of herbal medicine: India's opportunity. Current Med 2004; 86: 37-41.

[8]   Grover JK, Yadav S, Vats V. Medicinal plants of India with anti-diabetic potential. J Ethnopharmacol 2002; 81(1): 81-100.
[http://dx.doi.org/10.1016/S0378-8741(02)00059-4] [PMID: 12020931]

[9]   Newman DJ, Cragg GM. Natural products as sources of new drugs from 1981 to 2014. J Nat Prod 2016; 79(3): 629-61.
[http://dx.doi.org/10.1021/acs.jnatprod.5b01055] [PMID: 26852623]

[10]   Newman DJ, Cragg GM, Snader KM. Natural products in therapeutic. J Nat Prod 2003; 66: 1022.
[http://dx.doi.org/10.1021/np030096l] [PMID: 12880330]

[11]   Verpoorte R. Pharmacognosy in the new millennium: leadfinding and biotechnology. J Pharm Pharmacol 2000; 52(3): 253-62.
[http://dx.doi.org/10.1211/0022357001773931] [PMID: 10757412]

[12]   Shrager J. High throughput discovery: search and interpretation on the path to new drugs. Design for Science. Hillsdale, NJ, USA: Lawrence Erlbaum 2001; Vol. 11: pp. 325-48.

[13]   Farnsworth NR. The role of ethnopharmacology in drug development. Ciba Found Symp 1990; 154: 2-11.
[PMID: 2086037]

[14]   Farnsworth NR. Biological and phytochemical screening of plants. J Pharm Sci 1966; 55(3): 225-76.
[http://dx.doi.org/10.1002/jps.2600550302] [PMID: 5335471]

[15]   Wall ME, Wani MC. Camptothecin and taxol: from discovery to clinic. J Ethnopharmacol 1996; 51(1-3): 239-53.
[http://dx.doi.org/10.1016/0378-8741(95)01367-9] [PMID: 9213622]

[16]   Rastogi RP, Dhawan BN. Research on medicinal plants at the central drug research institute, Lucknow (India). Indian J Med Res 1982; 76 (Suppl.): 27-45.
[PMID: 6764455]

[17]   Cragg GM, Newman DJ. International collaboration in drug discovery and development from natural sources. Pure Appl Chem 2005; 77(11): 1923-42.
[http://dx.doi.org/10.1351/pac200577111923]

[18]   Harvey A. Strategies for discovering drugs from previously unexplored natural products. Drug Discov Today 2000; 5(7): 294-300.
[http://dx.doi.org/10.1016/S1359-6446(00)01511-7] [PMID: 10856912]

[19]   Baker JT, Borris RP, Carté B, *et al.* Natural product drug discovery and development: new perspectives on international collaboration. J Nat Prod 1995; 58(9): 1325-57.
[http://dx.doi.org/10.1021/np50123a003] [PMID: 7494142]

[20]   Mullard A. New drugs cost US$2.6 billion to develop. Nat Rev Drug Discov 2014; 13: 877.
[http://dx.doi.org/10.1038/nrd4507]

CHAPTER 2

Cultivation, Collection and Processing of Medicinal Plants

Omji Porwal[1,*], **Sachin Kumar Singh**[2], **Dinesh Kumar Patel**[3], **Saurabh Gupta**[4], **Rahul Tripathi**[5] and **Shankar Katekhaye**[6]

[1] *Department of Pharmacognosy, Faculty of Pharmacy, Tishk International University, Erbil, Kurdistan, Iraq*

[2] *School of Pharmaceutical Sciences, Lovely Professional University, Phagwara-144411, Punjab, India*

[3] *Faculty of Health Science, Shalom Institute of Health and Allied Sciences Sam Higginbottom University of Agriculture, Technology and Sciences (SHUATS)-State University (Formerly Allahabad Agriculture Institute) Naini, Allahabad, India*

[4] *Chitkara College of Pharmacy, Chitkara University, Chandigarh-patiala highway (NH-4), Rajpura Punjab 140401-India*

[5] *Medpharm Pharmaceutical Ltd. Guilford, United Kingdom*

[6] *Center for pharmaceutical Engineering Science University of Barford, Barford-BD71DP, United Kingdom*

Abstract: Nature has provided us better surroundings for the expansion and development of medicinal plants for thousands of years. Medicinal values of plants date back to ancient times on belief of its safety and economic value. Even in today's scenario, about 80% of the globe population primarily depends on the alternative system of medicines for their foremost healthcare requisite. Plants contain different types of secondary metabolites also called bioactive components of the plants responsible for their medicinal value in nature. Scientific cultivation permits the applying of contemporary technological aspects like mutation, polyploidy and hybridization for the development of a better amount of secondary metabolites from the plants and their byproducts. Cultivation, collection and preservations of medicinal plants need simple techniques that preserve the medicinal values of natural products. Pharmacological activities of medicinal and aromatic plants are mainly depending upon the presence of various bioactive phytochemicals like alkaloids, glycosides, tannins, resins, volatile oil, *etc.* Growth and development of medicinal plants and their secondary metabolites are mainly influenced by the physical surroundings, sunlight, temperature, rainfall, and nature of the soil. Seasonal variation and geographical region can also affect the quality of medicinal and aromatic plants as the concentration of bioactive constituent could be changed through natural factors. In the present book

* **Corresponding author Omji Porwal:** Department of Pharmacognosy, Faculty of pharmacy, Tishk International University, Erbil, Kurdistan Region, Iraq; Email:omji.porwal@tiu.edu.iq

Javed Ahmad and Javed Ahamad (Ed.)

chapter, we have discussed all the important information needed for the cultivation, collection and processing of medicinal and aromatic plants that affect the quality of medicinal plants.

Keywords : Cultivation, Collection, Drying, Harvesting, Medicinal Plants, Plant Growth Hormones.

1. IMPORTANCE OF MEDICINAL PLANTS

The crude drug that reaches the market and pharmaceutical industry must have some basic characteristics and quantity of active constituents for their claim therapeutic potential. Cultivation produces a quality of plants, increases secondary metabolite concentration, generates hybrids that produce specific phytoconstituents, ensures regular supply of crude drugs and also leads industrialization, *etc*. The gathering of crude medicine from cultivated plants provides a higher yield and therapeutic quality. Medicinal plants require sunny, aerated places sheltered from gale and late winter frosts. The soil must be fertile and consist of the required amounts of Na, P, Cu, alloy, organic and other essential elements for the better growth of medicinal and aromatic plants. Continuation of the farming structure has become a vital affair throughout the globe. A large number of the viable matter is related to the quality and time-dependent changes in the soil [1]. It is well known that in-depth cultivation has led to a swift rebuff in organic matter and nutrient levels besides affecting the physical things of clay [1]. However, the management practices with organic materials influence agricultural properties by the physical, chemical and biological properties of clay [2]. The implementation of organic amendments has long been recognized as an efficient suggestion for the improvement in the structure and fertility of the soil [3]. Increasing the microorganism diversity, activity, population and moisture-holding capability of soils also improve crop yield [4].

2. CULTIVATION OF MEDICINAL PLANTS

The demand for medicinal and aromatic plants has been increased in the market due to its better medicinal value and pharmacological activity that's why we need better care of medical care and mechanical management. If no scientific method of cultivation is available, then ancient strategies of cultivation should be followed. Otherwise, there is a need to develop a way of cultivation through scientific studies. The principles of agriculture practices together with appropriate rotation step with environmental suitableness, tailored to plant cultivation as per source needs. Conversation Agriculture (CA) capability ought to become behind where applicable, exceptionally builds up of fertile matter and conversation of soil humidness.

2.1. Method of Propagation

2.1.1. Sexual or Seed Propagation

Cultivation of medicinal plants by sexual propagation is by spreading or sowing seeds in suitable soil. Seeds are either shown by the dibbling method, in which the seeds of average size and weight are available, they are sown by placing in holes eg, fennel, coriander, *etc.*, or by the broadcasting method and this method is more applicable in case of the small size seeds. In this method, the seeds are scattered freely in well-prepared soil for cultivation, *e.g.* Isapgol linseed and sesame.

2.1.2. Asexual or Vegetative Propagation

In the case of the asexual method of vegetative propagation, the vegetative part of a plant, such as a stem or a root, is placed in such an environment that it develops into a new plant. The advantages of asexual propagation are there is no variation between the plant grown and plant from which it is grown. Seedlings of fruits can only be propagated vegetatively (*e.g.* Grapes, pomegranates and lemon), plant start bearing earlier as compared to seedling trees, budding or grafting encourages disease resistance varieties of plants, and inferior varieties can be overlooked. Vegetative propagation is done by sowing various parts of the plants in well-prepared soil. The following are examples of vegetative propagation:

Bulbs: squill, garlic

Corms: colchicum, saffron

Tubers: jalap, potato

Rhizomes: ginger, turmeric

Runners: peppermint

Suckers: mint, pineapple, banana, *etc.*

3. FACTORS AFFECTING CULTIVATION

Farming of medicinal and aromatic plants takes cognizance of plant habits and climatic requirements for their favourable growth. The factor which affects the cultivation of plants is listed below *i.e.* soil, altitude, temperature and humidity, rainfall or irrigation, fertilizers, pests and pest control.

3.1. Soil

The soil is outlined as a surface layer of the planet, fashioned by the eroding of rocks. The soil is made as a result of the amalgamation deed of weather strands like plants and microorganisms. The soil must contain an acceptable amount of nutrients, organic matter and alternative parts. Best soil nick, together with soil effluent, wet holding, fertility and pH are set as per the needs of the chosen curative plant. The use of compost is usually crucial to get good yields of medicinal plants. Soil influences seed to sprout, the potentiality of the plant to stay bolt upright form, vigour, and woodiness of the stem, depth of scheme, and range of flowers on a plan. Soils are of various types such as Clay, Loamy, Silt loam, Sandy loam, Sandy soil and Chalky soil.

Clay soils: Clay Particle is incredibly tiny. These match along terribly closely and thus, leave little or no pore house. These areas get crammed up with water terribly simply. Hence, the clay soil becomes quickly wet. Such soil has not much air; therefore, the plants growing in these soils aren't ready to absorb water. This soil is referred to as physiologically dry soil.

Sandy soil: Sand particles are big (0.02-02 mm) sized. These leave massive pore areas that do not have capillarity and so, water is not maintained by them. Most of the water is quickly drained off and reaches deep into the soil. As a result, roots unfold and additionally reach an excellent depth. The sandy soil is poor in nutrient elements; is less fertile and Plants rising in this soil have less dry mass.

Loam soil: It contains a mixture of clay and silt. It is incredibly helpful for the growth of plants. It is fertile and offers nutrients in enough amounts required for proper and diligent growth of plants. It has high water retention capability. The plants rising in this soil are vigorous and have a terribly high weight.

Silt loam: Silt soil is taken into account to be the foremost fertile because it contains an additional quantity of organic substances than other soil.

Sandy loam: It is a mixture of silt and clay.

3.2. Altitude, Temperature and Humidity

Climate factors, for instance, day duration, rainfall and temperature, considerably influence the physical, chemical and biological standard of medicinal plants. The period of daylight, average rainfall, minimal average temperature, including day-time and night duration temperature variations, additionally impact the biochemical pursuit of the plant.

3.3. Rainfall and Irrigation

Most of the plants need either proper arrangement for irrigation or sufficient rainfall for their favourable growth and development. Irrigation and drainage should be controlled and administered in accordance with the wants of the individual curative plant taxa throughout its various stages of rising. Water used for irrigation purpose ought to benefit native, regional and/or national quality standards. Supervision should be exercised to confirm that the curative plants under cultivation with sufficient required watered. Aloe and acacia are example of such xerophytes plant which do not requires irrigation or rainfall and its added advantage to cultivate such medicinal plant.

3.4. Fertilizers

A fertilizer is a mixture of organic and inorganic material unitized to increased soil fertility. There are various kinds of fertilizers.

Biotic origin fertilizer: Soil is generally poor in fertile organic matter and nitrogenous substances. This stuff of biological origin is utilised as fertiliser only if these can provide the elements required.

Green leaves manures: Manure is fertile material that is mixed with clay. These furnish most of the essential nutrients required by the curative plants. This leads to a rise in crop productivity.

Farmyard manure: This is a combination of live stock muck and remaining unutilised elements and husk and plants stalk fed to live stock.

Composite manure: This consists of a combination of delayed rotten and unutilised components of flora and fauna.

Green manure: This manure is non-woody crop ploughed beneath mixture with the soil whereas still inexperienced counterpoint the soil. The plants utilised as manure are typically fast growing. This is a nice mixture of organic as well as nitrogen component to the soil. It conjointly forms a protecting soil cowl that checks erosion and natural process. Due to this way curative plant mass will increase by 30-50%.

Bio- fertilizer: It is a outline as biologically active product of microorganism, alga and fungi that helps in delivering nutrient when applied to the soil. These principally embrace Nitrogen adjusting bio-organisms. Some of the Bio-fertilizer is Legume- bacteria genus mutualism, *Azolla-anabaena* mutualism, non-symbiotic microorganism, a not secure coalition of nitrogen adjusting bio-organism, *Eubacteria* that is a cynobacteria, a heterogeneous group of prokaryotic, principally photosynthetic organism.

Chemical fertilizers: Nitrogen, phosphorous, potassium, calcium, magnesium and sulphur are used as macronutrients; and iron, manganese, zinc, boron, copper, molybdenum, carbon, oxygen are used as micronutrients.

3.5. Pest and Pest Management

Pest is an undesired animal or plant species and pesticides are synthetically acquire from chemical and natural origin and effectual in small concentrations against pests. Different types of insects convey serious illness, such as malaria and typhus. Some insects demolish or cause heavy harm to valuable crops, such as *Zea mays, Gossypium, Triticum aestivum* and *Oryza sativa.* Other common pests include bacteria, fungi, *Rattus rattus* and such weeds as *Ambrosia artemisiiflora* and *Toxicodendron radicans.* An understanding of genesis of pest status is important in the design and execution of pest control strategies incorporating the substance of natural origin. Worldwide, the traditional pesticide represents the huge business in which the greater parts of the synthetic pesticides are for agriculture or other purposes.

3.5.1. Methods of Pest Control

3.5.1.1. Natural Controls

The natural world is full of the example of prey predator associations. Each and every pest is more or less hamper in its rise by other rapacious organisms. Parasitic pests, predators and the illness caused by the organism are usually the most important reason in natural way of insect controls. As the use of specific pesticides against a major pest on a crop might lead to a serious outbreak of a secondary pest due to the demolition of natural foe, which may lead to an upset in the balance between destructive and useful insects. Topographical influence of the seasonal changes such as hot-cold weather, rainfall, soil, atmospheric moisture and other climatic factors also show their impact on insects and their entertainer. Nevertheless in peculiar to the tropics, pleasant and frost climates, the pest sway methods are generally modify accordingly to the topographic surroundings.

3.5.1.2. Artificial Control

Artificial controls of pest have been start by human. Artificial control can be classified as agriculture, chemical and biological controls as discussed below.

3.5.1.3. Machine-like Mechanical Control

It employs self labour as well as mechanical devices for group or destruction of pest. Proficiency, such as handpicking, trimming, catching and blazing is employed for the knocking down of eggs, larvae, pupae and adult insects.

3.5.1.4. Agricultural Control

Agricultural control is the aged in its strategy. Deep plugging for the elimination of weeds and early stages of insects, follow one another crop rotation or changing environmental factor are some that cause to barrier of the life circle of pests. Nowadays latest modernised plant reproducing skills like mixing of good gene, control change in haploid set of chromosome, plant have more than two pair set of homologues chromosome and biotechnological betray are significantly used for the production of pest resistant taxa.

3.5.1.5. Chemical Controls

Chemical synthetic elements are the greatly used pesticides for the pest management all over the word. Such pesticides are used for the aim of killing pest for protecting curative plants, fauna or other belongings hostile to the strike of the pest. Insect impervious, attractants, fumigants like substance are utilised for killing bugs, ticks, and disinfectant elements which apply radioactive isotopes or chemicals. New groups of substance called a insect growth regulator (IGR), pesticides or bio insecticides be made up of the natural substance already available same in the insects that manage their growths. For example, 1-methyl (E,E)-11 methoxy-3,7,11-trimethyl-2,4-dodecadienoate also known as Altosid, ZR-515, Minex, that is a juvenile hormone avert the cocoon stage which grow the generative fully grown adults. Due to this way, larvae reproduce larger repeatedly and in due course die. Bio pesticides of this type are most precise for their noxiously action and welfare.

4. ROLE OF PLANT GROWTH REGULATORS

In the growing and maturing phase of medicinal plants are controlled by diversity of chemical compounds that are known as plants growth hormones. Specific five types of plants growth hormones are well accepted; they are the auxins (compounds with aromatic ring and carboxylic acid group), gibberellins (tetracyclic diterpene acids, usually synthesized by terpenoid pathway in plastid), cytokinins (adenine based structure compound), abscisic acid and its derivates, and ethylene. These compounds are of globe wide dispersal actually, take place entirely in higher plants. Plant growth regulators peculiar in their deed, and agile in extremely low quantity, and synchronize cell growth, biological operation, cell disparity, organogenesis, oldness, and dormancy. Their movement is maybe successive. Different hormones concerned with bloom formation and duplication, still yet uncharacterised, have collectively been predict. In spite of the first enthusiasm for analysis on drug improvement of hormones applied to medicinal crops.

4.1. Auxins

Auxin is a general term used to indicate substances that promote elongation of coleoptile tissues. Auxins were first studied in 1928 the Dutch botanist Frits Warmolt as well as other Dutch workers isolated two growth regulating substances such as auxin-a and auxin-b, acquire from human urine and cereal derivatives, respectively. They later noted that these had indistinguishable characteristics to Indole -3- acetic acid (IAA), the compound now accepted as the vital auxin. Several similar substances which are prospective parent of indole acetic acid have also been describe as natural products such as indole acetaldehyde, indole acetonitrile, and indole pyruvic acid from different plant origin. These all compounds and IAA are all originate, in the plants, from tryptophan amino acids.

4.2. Gibberellins

They are a class of endogenous plant growth regulators and at present over 50 gibberellins are known. These are cluster of plant growth regulators and were discovered by Japanese scientist in 1926 from *Oryza sativa*. Later, Yabuta and Hayashi isolated a crystalline specimen of the active compound as 'gibberellin'. Several gibberellins were identified from plant sources, and these plant regulators currently famed as Gibbrelic acid -1(GA-1), GA2, and GA3 unremarkably accepted as main gibberellin. The primary sensible manifestation that gibberellins actually subsist in higher plants came with West and Phinney's observations in

1956, that the liquid generative structure of the wild cucumber (*Echinocytis macrocarpa*) was in particular affluent in material have the gibberellins like action and Radley's report of a substance from *Pisum sativum* shoots showing as gibberellins on paper chromatograms [5].

4.3. Cytokinins

Cytokinins are either natural (zeatin) or synthetic (kinetin) compounds with significant growth regulating activities. They are different from auxins and gibberellins, as these are involved for mostly for cell expansion and cell growth procedure. Cytokinins are different compounds that have peculiar biological activity (*e.g.* Cytokinins). The German plant researcher Haberlandt in 1913 has focused that vascular tissues hold soluble compounds able of encouraging biological action in parenchymatous cells of injured solanum *tuberosum*.

4.4. Abscisic Acid

Natural growth inhibitors are found in plants and influence bud opening, seed development and happening of dormancy. One such compounds, abscisic acid (2Z, 4E)-5-[(1S)-1-hydroxy-2,6,6-trimethyl-4-oxocyclohex-2-en-1-yl]-3-methyl penta-2,4-dienoic acid was isolated and standardised in 1965. Abscisic acid isolated from the fungus *Cenospora rosicola* [6]. The structural resemblance of abscisic acid (ABA) to the carotenoids reminded research on the correlation of these two groups of compounds. It has now been reveal that few xanthophylls, particularly violaxanthin (a natural xanthophylls pigment with an orange colour biosynthesized from zeaxanthin by epoxidation), produce a reproductive inhibitor or on facing to sun light. Confirmation has now gather in favour of an indirect 'apocarotenoid' channel for ABA origin, the most resemblance pre-cleavage forerunner being *9'-* cis-neoxanthin and 9- cis-violaxanthin which cleavage over the 11, 12 (11', 12') double bond to make xanthoxin which in plant tissues is willingly modify in to ABA [7].

4.5. Ethylene

It has been investigated for ancient times that ethylene persuade growth responses in plants, and in 1932 it was revealed that the ethylene emit by stored apples reticent the growth of *solanum tuberosum* shoots surround with them. It has a part in fruit come to maturity. Ethylene biosynthesized in the plant form S-adenosyl methionine *via* the intermediate 1-aminocyclopropane-1-carboxylic acid (ACC). The genetic code for ACC synthase has been genetically similar form tomato squash [8]. One biochemical activity of ethylene is the initiation of the *de novo* synthesis and emission of cell wall dissolving enzymes same as cellulose during leaf abscission and fruit repining process. In the cell sap, at pH values above 4.0, it is dilapidated into ethylene and phosphate even at small amount ethylene has been shown to greater the concentration of glycosides in *Cassia angustifolia*.

4.6. Other Growth Regulators

In inclusion to the well known plant growth regulators and inhibitors compounds explore here, a great number of other substances have been isolated from natural origins which they may be influence plant growth drastically. Few are globally dispersed and others are of cramped in origin. Thus, these compounds may be act at many different specific areas along the growth regulatory process. Compounds comprise aliphatic and aromatic carboxylic acids, phenolic and natural compounds, salicylate, polyamines, S and N hetrocyclic compounds, consists alkaloids nitrogenous compounds and terpenes volatile unsaturated hydrocarbon substance. Sweet flag from acoraceae generates a number of sesquiterpenes, a class of three isoprene units having the skeltel structures of cadinane, acorane and eudesmane responsible for inhibiting the sprout of lettuce seeds [9]. A new class of plants growth regulators known as brassinosteroides (a class of polyhydroxylated steroidal phytoharmones with similar structure to animals) is found in the seeds, pollens, galls, leaves, flower buds, and shoots of a considerable range of plants. Among them 40 of such substances are now widely known; they encourage cell enlargement and cell division and impact genetic utterance and nucleic acid metabolism at the molecular extent [10].

5. ORGANIC FARMING

Organic farming ameliorates the standard of plant existence, maintains the organic miscellany, refine the soil composition and equitable the soil inhabiting microorganism in the absence of artificial chemicals. The concept and procedures are followed as the main principals of the international federation of organic agricultural movements (IFOAM, 2007), which are: (1) Making of ample top grade and nutritious food, (2) organic cultivation, priestly and untamed reap systems should fix the cycles and ecological stability in nature and should be tailored to mother states, ecology, culture, and scale, (3) Balance of natural soil fertility, (4) load ought to be lessen by new method, reprocess and systematic control of materials and energy in order to continue and ameliorate environmental calibre and conserve natural assets, (5) it should furnish everyone engaged with a good standard of life, and come up with to food sovereignty and depletion of paucity, (6) Professionals of agricultural can amplify efficient planning and grow productivity, but this should not be at chance of health and comfort, and as a result and detrimental act should be ceased [11].

6. COLLECTION OF MEDICINAL PLANTS

No matter what type of the crude drug and area of collection, there cannot be two opinions that the drugs are collected suitably when they contain maximum quantity of secondary plant metabolites. The collection of medicinal plant affected by few important things as: weather of the collected plant, plant age, daily session sunlight windy, and the phase of the physical growth of the plant part utilised [12]. The collection factors influence quality and quantity of the potent active component of plants: weather of the collected plant for example the leaves of Mentha, used for culinary propose, Eucalyptus species, a cash crop & Spearmint leave, used for memory enhancer during spring season contain a high content of volatile oils, while during hot & in cold weather the content of these oils become lessen. The medicinal plant age for examples cinchona tree species from rubiaceae have high amount of the alkaloid Quinine, a medication used to treat malaria and baesiosis and Cinchonine, antipyretic properties compound in their barks at their early age about 6 to 9 years old. The stage of Physiological development of medicinal plant used: for examples the leaves of (Digitalis, Tobacco & Senna) that are accumulate when they are in complete physiological maturity phase and the seeds of black cumin (*Nigella sativa*) are collected when they are white & black in colour.

7. HARVESTING OF MEDICINAL PLANTS

Harvesting is an important operation in cultivation technology, as it reflects upon economic aspects of the crude drugs. An important point which needs attention over here is the kind of drug to be harvested and the standard quality which it requires to attain. Medicinal plants ought to be harvested throughout the optimum weather or interval of time to confirm the assembly of curative plant stuff and end herb product of the simplest doable standard. The interval of harvesting based on the natural object to be utilised. Careful statistics regarding the suitable temporal arrangement of harvest is commonly obtainable in national pharmacopeia, printed authentic literature, latest official monographs, and vital reference books. Still, it is standard that the content of bioactive phytochemical depends with the phase of plant maturity. The simplest time for harvest ought to be determined in keeping with the standard amount of bioactive constituents instead of the full vegetative quantity of the focused curative plants. Throughout harvesting keep caution that no unwanted matter, weeds or noxious plants are assorted with the reap plant materials [13].

Curative plants ought to be harvested underneath the simplest doable states, keep away from condensation, rain or abnormally more wetness. Cutting tools, harvesters, and different apparatus ought to be washed and modify to contamination from soil and different materials. The harvested rough curative plant stuffs ought to be shift quickly in good, withered places. Harvested plant can be transferred in clean vessel, dry pouches, caravan, hoppers or different airy vessels and shift to the process supplying. All vessels used at harvest ought to be unbroken clean and free from foreign matter by accidently harvested curative plants and different contamination. Once vessels are not in function, they must be in good dry place states, in shielded section from insects, rodents, birds and different pest. Any machine injury or press down of the raw medicinal plant materials, as a result, as an example, of overfilling luggage avoided. Rotten medicinal plant materials ought to be known and discarded throughout harvest, post-harvest inspections, and process, so as to avoid microorganism contamination and degrade of raw medicinal plant material. It is compulsory to famous curative and aromatic medicinal plant in order to restore some of the traditional and economic medicinal plants [14, 15].

8. DRYING OF MEDICINAL PLANTS

It is very important to process properly medicinal drug before send to market. Drying is a step by which we preserve medicinal drug for long time with its pharmaceutical grace. As per medicinal drug origin source either animal or plant and its chemical nature help us to select various operations for their proper processing. Removal of sufficient moisture content from drug and maintain its standard and quality is also a necessary step of drying as well as this step also give no chance for growth of microorganism. Drying facilitate pulverizing and grinding as per need of finished product and inhibits partially enzymatic reactions too. In certain drugs, some specific procedure followed to achieve specific quality, *e.g.* fermentation in case of *Cinnamomum zeylanicum* bark and gentian roots [16]. The section and cutting into small pieces is done to enhance drying, as in case of *Glycyrrhiza glabra, Drimia maritima* and *Jateorhiza palmata*. The blooms are dried in shade so as to hold their colour and volatile oil content. Drying can be done in two ways, either by natural or artificial drying.

8.1. Natural Drying

Natural drying can be achieved by direct sun-light or shade. Mainly we preferred shade drying because it helps to retain its natural colour of the drug (*e.g.* digitalis, clove, senna) and the volatile principles of the drug (*e.g.* peppermint). We can also dry drug directly if it quite stable to the temperature and sunlight (*e.g.* gum acacia, seeds and fruits).

8.2. Artificial Drying

Artificial drying means if we used an oven; *i.e.* tray- dryers, vacuum dryer and spray dryers.

8.2.1. Tray Drying

If the drugs without volatile oils and completely stable to heat or which require deactivation of enzymes, then tray dryers used for drying. In tray drying hot air of the specific temperature is flow through the dryers and this make easy the removal of moisture content of the drugs (*e.g.* belladonna roots, cinchona bark, tea and raspberry leaves and gums are dried by this method).

8.2.2. Vacuum Drying

Tannic acid and digitalis leaves are sensitive to higher temperature thus used vacuum for drying.

8.2.3. Spray Drying

Few drugs which are highly reactive to atmospheric conditions and temperature are dried by spray-drying process. Papaya latex, pectin and tannin dried by this way [13].

9. GARBLING OF MEDICINAL PRODUCTS

The next step within the preparation of a crude drug for the market after drying is garbling. In this method foreign mater such as sand, dirt and foreign organic substance are separate from crude drugs. If the irrelevant matter is permit in crude medicine, the quality of drug surfers and probably, it fail pharmacopoeial limits. Excessive stems just in case of herbaceous plant. Medicine plant composes rhizomes got to be removed meticulously from roots and rootlets and additionally stem base items of iron should be removed with the magnet. Items of bark ought to be removed by peeling as in gum acacia.

10. PACKING OF MEDICINAL PRODUCTS

Well processed curative plant materials ought to be wrapping promptly to avert deterioration of the crude drugs and to protect in case of superfluous exposure to potential microbes strikes and various sources of contamination. Constant in-process internal authority measures ought to be applying to remove substandard materials, contaminants and unwanted matter before and through the ultimate phase of packaging. Processed curative plant stuff ought to be packaged in clean, dry boxes, luggage or different vessels in accordance with customised demand, requirement and national and/or regional laws of the manufacturer and consequently the end-user nation. Medicinal plant packaging material ought to be non-polluting, clean, dry and good condition and will change to the quality. Rigid containers ought to be used for fragile medicinal plant materials [12].

However the packaging used ought to be organised by the provider and client. Recycle wrapping stuff like jutes bag and mesh luggage ought to be cleansed (sterilize) and totally dried before reprocess, therefore to keep away foreign material by previous drug material. All wrapping stuff ought to be kept in a pest free dry clean environment. To avoided confusion medicinal plant drug material should be well labelled to the packaging with clear indication about botanical name, biological source, plant structure its assortment site, dates name of grower, collector and processor with its quantity. Additional label about its standard and quality approval should be with various required national and/or regional will give extra authentic advantage of medicinal drug plant. Official records ought to be unbroken with batch packaging and it will embrace the merchandise name, origin of place, batch scale, mass, assignment range with date. The records should be maintained as per various national and international and regional agencies authorities for their rules and regulation.

11. STORAGE AND PRESERVATION OF MEDICINAL PLANTS

The large-scale storage of medication may be a significant endeavour. However *Cascara sagrada* barks on long storage, though usually ineluctable, is not counselled medication like Cannabis plant and *Sarsaparilla officinalis* decline even once rigorously keep. Literature survey shows that the content of taxol in *Taxus baccata* leaves and extracts go low 30-40% after challenging in temperature up to one year even though storage in a deep freeze and direct daylight [16]. Similarly, the alkamides a lipophilic constitutes of the popular immunity enhancer herb eastern purple cone flower decline quickly on preservation [17]. It has been reported that drying has little effect on the number of alkamides, storage for 64 weeks at 24°C produces an 80% moisture, as compared to if drugs stored in the usual containers-sacks, bales, wooden cases, cardboard boxes, and paper bags-reabsorb about 10-12% moisture. Starch, acacia gum and others must have control moisture content as per standard BP and European Pharmacopoeia. The conjoint outcome of moisture and temperature on wetness and the succeeding water-condensation when the decrease in temperature must be mind in drug storage. Drugs such as Digitalis and Cannabis plant may lose a considerable part of their activity if we go air drying. Stored those sealed containers with a dehydrating agent. Originally grown curative plant stuff should be preserved and transfer individually or in a manner that make sure their specific unity. Suitable security measures should be put to the preservation and transfer of medicinal plant stuff that are potentially noxious or lethal [13].

CONCLUDING REMARKS

The cultural price attributed to medicinal plants can be used as associate argument to support the conservation of diversity. However, such cultural values are not essentially identical for wild and cultivated plants, and it is necessary to tell apart between cultural aspects regarding the employment of the plants and cultural values relating to their cultivation. Traditional and Ayurvedic practitioners use medicinal plants and their parts as raw materials for the preparation of various types of traditional medicinal formulations. Scientifically validated process of medicinal and aromatic plant preparation has not developed adequately in the history and the developed modern medicine. Majorly the traditional method has been used in the Herbal manufacturing and processing unit and still very limited update have been done. A distinct project may be taken up in order to familiarize some of the medicinal drug crop, which is in great call from the cosmetic neutraceutical, food and pharmaceutical industry. Such projects will go a long way in reward the farmers to tackle professional growth of medicinal and aromatic crops. The scientific farming development, harvesting and processing of medicinal plants is the essential requirement of today's herbal drug industry in resuming productive and authentic standard drugs to the humanity.

ABBREVIATIONS

ABA   Abscisic acid

ACC   1-Aminocyclopropane-1-carboxylic acid

CA   Conservation Agriculture

FRLHT Foundation for revitalisation of local health traditions

GAP   Good Agricultural Practices

GA   Gibberellic acid

IFOAM International federation of organic agriculture

IAA   Indole- 3-acetic acid

MAPs   Medicative and aromatic plants

OA   Organic agriculture

WHO   World Health Organization

CONSENT FOR PUBLICATION

Not applicable.

CONFLICT OF INTEREST

The author(s) confirms that there is no conflict of interest.

ACKNOWLEDGEMENTS

Authors indebted acknowledge Dr. Esra Tariq Anwer , Dr. Muath sheet Mohmamd Ameen the facilities provided by Faculty of Pharmacy, Tishk International University, Erbil, Kurdistan Region, Iraq.

REFERENCES

[1]   Karlen DL, Mausbach MJ, Doran JW, Cline RG, Harries RF, Schuman GE. Soil quality: a concept, definition and framework for evaluation. Soil Sci Soc Am J 1997; 61: 4-10.
        [http://dx.doi.org/10.2136/sssaj1997.03615995006100010001x]

[2]   Saha S, Mina BL, Gopinath KA, Kundu S, Gupta HS. Relative changes in phosphatase activities as influenced by source and application rate of organic composts in field crops. Bioresour Technol 2008; 99(6): 1750-7.
        [http://dx.doi.org/10.1016/j.biortech.2007.03.049] [PMID: 17507214]

[3]   Follet R, Donahue R, Murphy L. Soil and soil amendments. New Jersey: Prentice-Hall, Inc. 1981.

[4]   Frederickson J, Butt KR, Morris MR, Daniel C. Combining vermiculture with green waste composting system. Soil Biol Biochem 1997; 29: 725-30.
        [http://dx.doi.org/10.1016/S0038-0717(96)00025-9]

[5]   Wynne G, Mander LN, Goto N, Yamane H, Omori T. Gibberellin A117 methyl ester, a new antheridiogen from *Lygodium circinnatum*. Phytochemistry 1998; 49(7): 1837-40.
        [http://dx.doi.org/10.1016/S0031-9422(98)00415-4]

[6]   Evans WC. Trease and Evans, Pharmacognosy. 16th ed., New York: Elsevier 2009.

[7]   Parry AD, Horgan R. Carotenoid metabolism and the biosynthesis of abscisic acid. Phytochemistry 1991; 30(3): 815-21.
        [http://dx.doi.org/10.1016/0031-9422(91)85258-2]

[8]   Klee H, Estelle M. Molecular genetic approaches to plant hormone biology. Annu Rev Plant Biol 1991; 42(1): 529-51.
        [http://dx.doi.org/10.1146/annurev.pp.42.060191.002525]

[9]   Nawamaki K, Kuroyanagi M. Sesquiterpenoids from *Acorus calamus* as germination inhibitors. Phytochemistry 1996; 43(6): 1175-82.
        [http://dx.doi.org/10.1016/S0031-9422(96)00401-3]

[10]   Khripach VA. Brassinosteroids, a New Class of Plant Hormone. San Diego: Academic Press 1999.

[11]   IFOAM (International Federation of Organic Agriculture Movements). The Organic Principles 2007.http://www.ifoam.org

[12]   World health organization WHO guidelines on good agricultural and collection practices (GACP) for medicinal plants, 2003.

[13]   Shah B, Seth AK. Test book of Pharmacognosy and Phytochemistry. Elsevier 2010.

[14] Government of India Report of the Task Force on Conservation and Sustainable Use of Medicinal Plants, Planning Commission, Govt of India, New Delhi 2000.

[15] Medicinal Plants of India: Guidelines for National Policy and Conservation Programmes, FRLHT, Bangalore 1997.

[16] Das B, Rao SP, Kashinatham A. Taxol content in the storage samples of the needles of Himalayan *Taxus baccata* and their extracts. Planta Med 1998; 64(1): 96.
[http://dx.doi.org/10.1055/s-2006-957383] [PMID: 9491774]

[17] Perry NB, van Klink JW, Burgess EJ, Parmenter GA. Alkamide levels in *Echinacea purpurea*: effects of processing, drying and storage. Planta Med 2000; 66(1): 54-6.
[http://dx.doi.org/10.1055/s-2000-11111] [PMID: 10705735]

CHAPTER 3

Extraction of Bioactive Phytochemicals

Javed Ahamad[1,*], **Naila Hassan Ali Alkefai**[2] and **Shehla Nasar Mir Najibullah**[3]

[1] *Department of Pharmacognosy, Faculty of Pharmacy, Tishk International University, Kurdistan Region, Erbil, Iraq*

[2] *Department of Pharmacognosy, Faculty of Pharmacy, University of Hafer Albatin, Hafer Albatin, KSA*

[3] *Department of Pharmacognosy, Faculty of Pharmacy, King Khalid University, Abha, KSA*

Abstract: The success of pharmacological or analytical study depends upon proper choice of the extraction method. As extraction process is the starting step in the evaluation of any herbal drug, hence it should be designed in such a way that the extracts contain maximum amount of desired secondary metabolites. Several classical extraction methods are used since ancient times, such as percolation, digestion, decoctions, and maceration. Due to the advancement in technology, several extraction techniques have been developed, such as ultrasound assisted extract, microwave assisted extraction, pressurized liquid extraction, supercritical fluid extract and enzyme assisted extraction. These extraction techniques provide samples for qualitative and quantitative analysis of the natural product. The extracts obtained from these extraction methods are also used for the isolation and characterization of bioactive natural products. This book chapter provides a comprehensive overview of a variety of classical and modern extraction methods used in drug discovery and development from the natural product.

Keywords: Bioactive Phytochemicals, Extraction, Isolation, Modern Extraction Methods, Natural Products, Secondary Metabolites.

1. INTRODUCTION

Extraction is the first step in obtaining desired bioactive phytochemicals from medicinal plants and it is defined as *"the separation medicinally active portions of plant and animal tissue using selective solvents by standard procedures"*. Medicinal plants and their bioactive natural compounds have records of use as food, cosmetics and medicine.

* **Corresponding author Dr. Javed Ahamad:** Department of Pharmacognosy, Faculty of Pharmacy, Tishk International University, Kurdistan Region, Erbil, Iraq; E-mails: jas.hamdard@gmail.com & javed.ahamad@tiu.edu.iq

More advanced and efficient extraction and separation techniques are required due to the increased demands of these phytochemicals from the industries. Many traditional or classical extraction methods have been used previously to extract bioactive phytochemicals such as maceration, percolation, digestion decoction, *etc.* In recent decades, certain modern extraction techniques have also been developed for the efficient extraction of natural products due to advances in technology. Even the advent of modern and sophisticated extraction techniques has not yet been found to be suitable for all forms of phytochemicals [1]. That is why, depending on the nature of crude drugs and the suitability of extraction techniques, we used specific methods for particular crude drugs [2, 3]. Medicinal plants are the largest source of bioactive phytochemicals in several conventional and modern medical practices, which are used traditionally as medicines. Medicinal plants containing essential oils are a major source of fragrances, flavors, cosmeceuticals and health beverages. Elevated temperature causes a detrimental effect on the chemical composition of essential oils for extraction. That is why special extraction methods are used to separate these compounds under low temperatures. Mostly medicinal plants are traded as such in bulk from many developing and underdeveloped countries for value-added in developed countries. The first step in adding value to the wealth of medicinal plants is to extract in the form of galenicals or dried extracts. Various types of herbal extracts, infusions, tinctures and herbal tea are commercially available in the market [4]. These preparations are also known as decoctions, fluid extracts, pilular extracts or powdered extract. The need to develop a standardized extraction procedure for crude drugs is to achieve the therapeutically desired portions and to eliminate unwanted materials by using a selective solvent treatment. The extracts thus obtained after standardized methods of extraction could be used as medicinal agents as such or incorporated in the finished dosage form such as tablets and capsules or used in further studies [5].

These extracts contain bioactive phytochemicals of medicinal plants belonging to different classes of secondary metabolites such as alkaloids, glycosides, terpenoids, flavonoids, tannins, resins, fixed oils, essential oils and lignans *etc.* In order to be used as modern drugs, extracts could be further processed by means of various isolation and purification techniques of bioactive phytochemicals such as counter current chromatography, flash chromatography, preparative HPLC, preparative TLC and preparative GC *etc.* The book chapter provides a comprehensive overview of a number of classical and modern extraction methods that are used in the production and development of herbal drugs.

2. STEPS INVOLVED IN THE EXTRACTION OF MEDICINAL PLANTS

Numerous new methods have been developed along with conventional methods, but so far, no single method is considered the standard for plant extraction of bioactive compounds. The qualitative and quantitative studies of bioactive compounds from plant materials depend mostly on choosing the proper method of extraction. The various steps involve the extraction of medicinal ingredients from plant materials, such as drying and grinding of plant materials, selection of suitable solvents, extraction, filtration, concentration and drying of the extract [6].

2.1. Drying and Grinding of Plant Materials

In most cases, before the place of work, plant material is dried in the atmosphere. It can be dried at room temperature or below 45 °C in the oven. If plant materials were left to stand for several days, compacted samples of fresh plant material with little air circulation could experience fungal infestation and fermentation at elevated temperatures. Well ventilated places and homogeneous material distribution should therefore be ensured. The equipment used for grinding plant materials is advanced mills, blenders, simple axes, scissors, grinders, or knives. When extracting thermolabile or volatile phytocompounds the milling stage may be omitted to avoid heat-generating losses during communition. The grinding process assists solvent penetration into the cellular structure of the plant tissues, thus helping to dissolve the secondary metabolites and increase extraction yields. Size reduction also maximizes the surface area, which in effect facilitates the transfer of mass of the active principle from the plant material to the solvent.

2.2. Selection of Suitable Solvents

Care should be taken to consider the solvents selected for extraction. The selected solvent should dissolve the under-study secondary metabolites, be easy to remove, and be inert, non-toxic and, not easily flammable. Solvents should be distilled if they are of low or unknown quality before use. Examples of solvents commonly used for extraction studies include water, ethanol, and methanol *etc*.

2.3. Extraction Process

The simplest extraction processes employed are organic solvent extraction; percolation, maceration, and extraction using a Soxhlet device; and water extraction; infusion, decoction, and distillation of steam. Extraction of plant materials nowadays by various modern or non-conventional techniques of extraction, such as ultrasonic-assisted extraction (UAE), microwave-assisted extraction (MAE), pressurized liquid extraction (PLE), and supercritical fluid extraction (SFE).

2.4. Filtration

The extract thus obtained is separated from the marc (exhausted plant material) by allowing it to drip through the inserted false bottom of the extractor, which is filled with a filter paper, into a holding tank. At the false bottom, the marc is retained and the extract is obtained in the holding tank. The extract is pumped from the holding tank into a sparkler filter for the removal of fine or colloidal particles from the extract.

2.5. Concentration

The enriched extract from the percolators or extractors, known as miscella, is fed into a wiped film evaporator where a densely concentrated extract is concentrated under vacuum. Nowadays, rota-evaporator is used frequently in pharmaceutical industries and laboratories for the concentration of thermolabile and heat-sensitive compounds such as flavonoids, polyphenols, and glycosides.

2.6. Drying of Extract

The condensed extract is subjected to spray drier at a controlled feed rate and temperature with a high-pressure pump, to get dry powder. The desired product particle size is obtained by regulating the chamber's internal temperature and by adjusting the pump speed. The dry powder is combined with the necessary diluents or excipients and blended in a double cone mixer to produce a powder that can be straightaway used for infilling of capsules or making tablets. In the pharmaceutical industry and laboratories, several other methods are used to dry extracts such as freeze-drying/lyophilization, rotary evaporation, air-drying, and oven drying [6].

3. FACTORS AFFECTING EXTRACTION PROCESS

The extraction of phytochemicals includes the following steps: (1) the solvent penetrates the solid matrix; (2) the solutes dissolve in the solvents; (3) the solvent is diffused out of the solid matrix; and (4) the solutes extracted are collected. Any invoice which enhances the diffusivity and solubility in the above steps will facilitate the extraction. The properties of the extraction solvents, the particle size of crude drugs the solvent-to-solid ratio, the extraction temperature, and extraction duration will affect the efficiency of extraction [6, 7]. Solvent plays a key role in natural product extraction. The polarity of solvents is an important parameter in the extraction process, since *"like dissolves like"* polar solvents used to extract polar drugs and non-polar solvents are used to extract non-polar drugs. Solvents should be selected based on safety, cost, and polarity for efficient extraction. The most common solvents used for the extraction of natural products are ethanol, methanol, and water. Temperature also plays a key role in the extraction process, as temperature increases, solubility increases, and diffusion. However, this too high temperature may cause the loss of solvents, as well as more possibilities for the degradation of thermolabile compounds. The particle size of crude plant material also affects the extraction yields. In the extraction of plant materials coarse to a fine powder is considered as better for efficient extraction. The extraction efficiency will be enhanced by fine powder due to the enhanced penetration and increase in surface area of the crude drug. Duration of extraction also plays an important role in increasing extraction yield, with an increase in extraction duration extraction efficiency increases up to certain levels after that it is not affecting. The longer extraction period due to the breakdown of phytochemicals causes negative effects on extraction efficiency. The amount of solvents also influences the yield of extraction, if the solvent to the solid ratio is higher the saturation of the solvents is lower and extraction is higher, but more solvents often require a long time for phytochemical extraction [4].

4. METHODS OF EXTRACTION

4.1. Classical Methods of Extraction

In classical methods of extraction, the polarity of solvents and application of heat and/or mixing plays an important role. The most common existing classical extraction techniques are percolation, digestion, decoctions, maceration, soxhlation, reflux extraction *etc.* Hydrodistillation using the Clevenger apparatus is used for the isolation of essential oils from aromatic medicinal plants. The infusion and digestion are not used frequently for the extraction of secondary metabolites in drug development [6].

4.1.1. Maceration

Maceration is used for the extraction of thermolabile herbal drugs. It is a simple method of extraction and does not require sophisticated equipments. The crude drugs in coarse powder form are kept in a stoppered container with suitable solvents for a period of time (usually 3 to 7 days) with vocational heating. After the desired time, the extracts are filtered and fresh solvents are added and again filtered. Both filtrates are combined and evaporated under vacuum. The major limitation of this method is that it requires a long time for extraction. Cujic *et al.*, studied the extraction of total phenols and anthocyanins from chokeberry fruits using the maceration technique [8]. Catechins were extracted from *Arbutus unedo* fruits by maceration, microwave, and ultrasonic methods and compared, the maceration method was found nearly equal to microwave-assisted extraction at low temperature [9].

4.1.2. Decoction

The decoction method of extraction is a very simple method of extraction; in this method, a defined weight of the powdered crude drug is boiled with a specified volume of water for a defined period. The extract is filtered and cooled for further use. This method of extraction is suitable for the extraction of water-soluble and heat stable natural products. The major disadvantage with decoction method are that it cannot be applied for the extraction of thermolabile drugs. Li *et al.*, studied the decoction-induced chemical transformation of ginsenosides in ginseng by UPLC-MS/MS [10]. Zhang *et al.*, studied the chemical transformation of flavonoid glycosides in a herbal formulation containing *Astragali radix* and *Angelicae sinensis radix* [11].

4.1.3. Percolation

Percolation is used frequently to prepare mother tinctures in homeopathic formulations. In this method of extraction, a powdered crude drug is first moistened and then kept in a percolator which is narrow, cone-shaped vessel open at both ends for a specified time (usually 6 to 21 days) in a suitable solvent. After the desired time of extraction, the extract is collected and the required volume is made with solvent. Percolation is more efficient than maceration, digestion, decoction, and infusion. The major limitation of this method is that it requires a long time for extraction. Zhang *et al.*, extracted fucoxanthin from *Undaria pinnatifida* by using the percolation and refluxing extraction method and he found that the percolation method yields are higher than the refluxing method [12].

4.1.4. Reflux Extraction

In this extraction method, coarse powders of drugs are refluxed with suitable solvents for 1 to 4 hrs. After extraction, the extract is filtered and concentrated under vacuum. Reflux extraction is a fast and simple method mostly applied for the extraction of heat-stable natural products. The main disadvantage of reflux extraction is that it cannot be used for the extraction of thermolabile drugs such as flavonoids, terpenes, and polyphenols *etc.* Kongkiatpaiboon *et al.,* studied the extraction of didehydrostemofoline from *Stemona collinsiae* by reflux extraction method, he reported higher efficiency in reflux extraction compared to soxhlation, maceration, and percolation [13]. Zhang *et al.,* studied the extraction of baicalin and puerarin from Chinese traditional medicine (TCM) by using reflux and decoction extraction methods, he found that the reflux method is better in extraction yield compared to the decoction method [14].

4.1.5. Soxhlet Extraction

Soxhlet method is the most common method used in Pharmacognosy laboratories for extraction of medicinal plants for samples required for isolation and characterization of moderately heat stable compounds such as alkaloids, resins, flavonoids, glycosides *etc.* for extraction of crude drugs in coarse powder form packed in Soxhlet apparition and extracted with organic solvents such as methanol, chloroform, petroleum ether, hexane *etc.* for a specified time (usually 6 to 9 hrs). After extraction, the extract is evaporated under vacuum and dried. The main advantage of this method are that it is continuous, fast, and requires fewer solvents compared to maceration, percolation, and decoction. The main disadvantage of this method is that it is not suitable for the extraction of thermolabile drugs. Wei *et al.,* reported a high yield of ursolic acid (38.21 mg/g) in a Chinese traditional medicine Cynomorium by the Soxhlet extraction method [15]. Chin *et al.,* studies the degradation of catechins in tea extracts using Soxhlet extraction at high temperatures [16].

4.1.6. Isolation of Essential Oils

Hydrodistillationmethod is the most common method used in laboratories for the isolation of essential or volatile oils. To isolate essential oils, fresh plant material is placed with water in the Clavenger apparatus and extracted for 6 to 8 hrs. After extraction, the volatile oil is collected in a graduated tube of Clavenger apparatus, is collected in closed glass vials and stored in a refrigerator at 4 °C. There are several other methods available for the extraction of essential oils such as supercritical fluid extraction, ecuelle, effleurage *etc.* Yahya and Yunus, found that the time taken to extract Patchouli essential oil obtained by the hydrodistillation method did not affect the quality [17]. Hamad *et al.,* performed isolation of essential oils by hydrodistillation method from *Lavandula angustifolia* and found camphor (13.58%) as major compound [18]. Naquvi *et al.,* isolated essential oils from the *Origanum vulgare* hydrodistillation method and he found carvacrol acetate (66.01%)as the major compound [19]. Ahamad *et al.*, isolated essential oil by hydrodistillation method from *Rosmarinus officinalis* leaves and found the verbenone (23.46%), 1,8-cineol (15.96%), α-pinene (12.10%), camphor (10.98%), and bornyl acetate (5.78%) as major components [20]. The authors also reported that *R. officinalis* essential oil causes inhibition of the α-glucosidase enzyme (IC$_{50}$ value 9.64±2.44μg/mL) and produces dose-dependant cytotoxicity against human breast adenocarcinoma MDA-MB-231cells (IC$_{50}$ value 59.35 μg/mL).

4.2. Modern Methods of Extraction

In recent decades, due to advancement in scientific technologies, several new extraction techniques emerged such as ultrasound-assisted extraction (UAE), microwave-assisted extraction (MAE), pressurized liquid extraction (PLE), supercritical fluid extraction (SFE), enzyme assisted extraction (EAE) *etc.* these advance and sophisticated extraction techniques are fast, need less solvents, reduce possible breakdown of natural products and environment friendly. Various modern techniques are summarized in Table **1** and the application of each extraction technique is presented in Table **2**.

Table 1. **Advantages of various extraction techniques in the extraction of bioactive natural products.**

Extraction Methods	Temperature	Time	Solvents	Solid to Solvent Ratio	Cost
Maceration	Room temperature	Long	Any solvent	High	Economical
Decoction	Under heat	Short	Water	High	Economical
Percolation	Room temperature	Long	Any solvent	High	Economical
Reflux extraction	Under heat	Short	Any solvent	Moderate	Economical
Soxhlation	Under heat	6 to 8 hrs	Organic solvents	Moderate	Economical
Hydrodistillation	Under heat	6 to 8 hrs	Water	Moderate	Economical
UAE	Low	10 to 60 minutes	Any solvent	Small	Moderate
MAE	Low	10 to 60 minutes	Any solvent	Small	Moderate
PLE	Low	Short	Any solvent	Small	Expensive
SFE	Low	Short	Supercritical fluid (CO$_2$), sometime ethanol as modifier	None or very small	Expensive
EAE	Room temperature or heated after enzyme treatment	Long	Any solvent	Moderate	Expensive

4.2.1. Ultrasound-Assisted Extraction (UAE)

In ultrasound-assisted extraction method, the powdered crude is kept in a stoppered conical flask with suitable solvents for a specified period (usually 10 to 60 minutes). After extraction, the drug is filtered and evaporated under a vacuum in rota-evaporator at low temperature. Ultrasound-assisted extraction method is suitable for the extraction of thermolabile herbal drugs, the main advantages of it are that it requires a short time for extraction, minimum quantity of solvents, is environment friendly, and gives higher extraction yield. It is considered as a green extraction technology as it requires very less amount of solvents and is environment friendly. In UAE method, ultrasonic energy (20 kHz to 100 MHz) assists extract by increasing the diffusion of solvents across the cell wall, and the ringing of the content with solvents with cell after breaking the walls [21 - 23]. Rostagno *et al.*, studied the extraction efficiency of isoflavone derivatives from soybean by UAE method using different times and solvents [24]. Yang and Zhang, developed and optimized ultrasonic extraction conditions for rutin and quercetin from *Euonymus alatus* [25]. Ultrasonic extraction is also applied for extraction vindoline, catharanthine and vinblastine from Vinca [26], anthocyanins and phenolics from grape peel [27, 28], phenol carboxylic acids, carnosic acid and rosmarinic acid from Rosmery [29]. This method is also utilized for extraction of phytosterols [30], saponins [31], flavonoids [23], and polysaccharides from plants [32]. The authors also developed and standardized UAE technique for extraction of swertiamarin a secoiridoid glycosides from aerial parts of *Enicostemma littorale* [7]; gymnemic acids from leaves of *Gymnema sylvestre* [33]; and charantin from fresh ripe fruits of *Momordica charantia* [5], and compared with Soxhlet extraction method. The UAE method was found about three-time more efficient in extracting swertiamarin, gymnemic acids, and charantin from respective plants compared to the Soxhlet extraction method.

4.2.2. Microwave-Assisted Extraction (MAE)

The microwave extraction technique is considered a green extraction technology because it requires a very less amount of organic solvents and is environment friendly. MAE utilizes microwave energy (300 MHz to 300 GHz) for assisting the extraction of bioactive natural compounds [34]. The major advantages of MAE are that it requires minimum amount of solvents and time, and also can be used for the extraction of heat-sensitive compounds. It is applied for extraction of caffeine and other polyphenols from green tea leaves [35], ginsenosides from ginseng roots [36], flavolignin and silybinin from milk thistle [37], guggolsterone, cinnamaldehyde and tannins from various medicinal plants [38], phenolic acids from bran and flour fractions of sorghum and maize [39], and flavonoids and phenolics from different plants [40].

4.2.3. Pressurized Liquid Extraction (PLE)

The pressurized liquid extraction method was developed and used by Richter *et al.*, in 1966. In this method of extraction, high pressure is maintained which helps in keeping solvents in liquid state even after its boiling point. At this state, solvent penetrate cells and tissues of crude drugs at higher rates and helps extraction. The main advantage of PLE are that it requires minimum amount of solvents and time [41]. This technique is applied for the extraction of several natural products such as isoflavones from soybeans [42], terpenoids and sterols from tobacco [43], phenolic compounds from *Petroselinum crispum* [44], lycorine and galanthamine from *Narcissus jonquilla* [45], and phenolics (for *e.g.* catechin, epicatechin gallate, caffeic acid, chlorogenic acid and myristin) from *Anatolia propolis* [46].

4.2.4. Supercritical Fluid Extraction (SFE)

The supercritical fluid extraction method is extensively applied for the extraction of thermolabile natural products specifically essential oils. SFE needs solvents in the supercritical states for the extraction of natural products. At the supercritical stage, fluid possesses gas like properties such as diffusion, viscosity, and surface tension; and liquid-like density, and salvation power. Carbon dioxide is considered as an ideal solvent for SFE. The critical temperature and pressure of CO_2 were 31 °C and 74 bars pressure. At a supercritical state, CO_2 offers the possibility to operate at moderate pressure and behaves as a liquid which penetrates the cells and tissues and assists extraction [47]. SFE offers quick extraction of thermolabile components of plants such as essential oils. SFE is widely utilized for the extraction of phytochemicals such as: purine alkaloids (caffeine, theobromine, and theophylline) from *Ilex paraguaryensis* [48], naringin a flavonoid from citrus [49], polyphenols, procyanidins, catechin and epicatechin from grape seed [50], and Vinca alkaloids [51].

4.2.5. Enzyme Assisted Extraction (EAE)

In this extraction method, the hydrolytic action of certain enzymes such as glucose oxidase, amyloglucosidase, hemicellulose, amylase, cellulase, pectinase, *etc.* facilitates extraction of bioactive molecules from raw plant materials. These enzymes cause the breakdown of phytochemicals and cellular structures and facilitate the extraction process. Recently, enzyme assisted extraction method is utilized for the extraction of several bioactive phytochemicals, some applications of this method are discussed in this section. Chen *et al.*, reported the extraction of polysaccharides from *Astragalas membranaceus* using various enzymes and reported that glucose oxidase shows a higher extraction yield [52]. Strati *et al.*, studied the extraction of carotenoid and lycopene from tomato waste using pectinase and cellulase enzymes and compared with non-enzyme treated solvent extraction, he found that the extraction yield is higher in enzyme-treated samples [53]. Liu *et al.*, studied extraction of chlorogenic acid from *Eucommia ulmoides* leaves using cellulase and ionic liquids, he found that the extraction yield greatly increased by enzyme treatment [54].

Table 2. Application of modern extraction methods in the extraction of natural products.

Extraction Method	Phytocompounds	Source	References
Ultrasound-assisted extraction (UAE)	Charantin	*Momordica charantia*	[5]
	Swertiamarin	*Enicostemma littorale*	[7]
	Gymnemic acids	*Gymnema sylvestre*	[33]
	Daidzin, genistin, glycitin and malonyl genistin	*Glycine max*	[24]
	Rutin and quercetin	*Euonymus alatus*	[25]
	Vindoline, catharanthine and vinblastine	*Catharanthus roseus*	[26]
	Anthocyanins and phenolic compounds	Grape peel	[27, 28]
	Phenolcarboxylic acids, carnosic acid and rosmarinic acid	*Rosmarinus officinalis*	[29]
Microwave-assisted extraction (MAE)	Polyphenols and caffeine	*Thea sinensis* (Green tea)	[35]
	Ginsenosides	*Panax ginseng*	[36]
	Flavolignin and silybinin	*Silybum marianum*	[37]
	E- and *Z*-guggolsterone, cinnamaldehyde and tannin from	Various plant sps.	[38]
Pressurized liquid extraction (PLE)	Isoflavones	*Glycine max* (soybean)	[42]
	Terpenoids and sterols	*Nicotiana tabacum* (Tobacco)	[43]
	Phenolic compounds	*Petroselinum crispum*	[44]
	Lycorine and galanthamine	*Narcissus jonquilla*	[45]
	Phenolic compounds	*Anatolia propolis*	[46]

(Table 2) cont.....

Supercritical fluid extraction (SFE)	Caffeine, theobromine, and theophylline	*Ilex paraguaryensis*	[48]
	Naringin	*Citrus* sps.	[49]
	Polyphenols, procyanidins, catechin and epicatechin	*Vitis vinifera*(Grape seed)	[50]
	Indolealkaloids (catharanthine)	*Catharanthus roseus*	[51]
Enzyme assisted extraction (EAE)	Polysaccharides	*Astragalas membranaceus*	[52]
	Carotenoid and lycopene	*Solanum lycopersicum*(tomato)	[53]
	Chlorogenic acid	*Eucommia ulmoides*	[54]

5. CASE STUDIES: BIOACTIVE PHYTOCHEMICAL ISOLATION AND PURIFICATION

5.1. Piperine

Piperine (Fig. **1**) is obtained from the dried, unripe fruits of *Piper nigrum* (Piperaceae). Piperine occurs as a colourless or slightly yellowish crystal having a melting point 136-138˚C. Initially, tasteless but later produces a burning sensation. It is practically insoluble in water. Piperine gives maximum absorption at 245 nm in UV spectrum. Pepper was once employed in the treatment of gonorrhoea and chronic bronchitis. Pepper in large quantities used as a condiment.

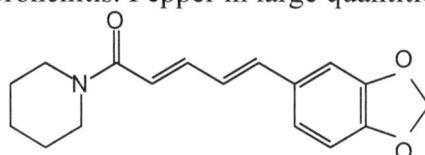

Piperine

Fig. (1). Chemical structure of Piperine.

5.2. Piperine Isolation

1. Approximately 20 g of black pepper powder is extracted with 250 ml of ethanol (95%) in the Soxhlet apparatus for 6 hr.
2. The solution is filtered and the filtrate concentrated on a hot water bath under reduced pressure using a rotary evaporator.
3. 20 ml of 10% alcoholic KOH solution is added to the concentrated filtrate with constant stirring.
4. Filter the solution and kept it overnight. Slightly yellowish crystals of piperine separate out.
5. Recrystallize it with a mixture of acetone and hexane (3:2).

5.3. Quinine

Quinine (Fig. **2**) is obtained from the dried bark of *Cinchona officinalis, C. succirubra* and other species of *Cinchona* (Rubiaceae). Quinine is an important quinoline alkaloid of cinchona bark. It is a stereoisomer of quinidine and has antimalarial property. Quinine is mainly used for the treatment of malaria.

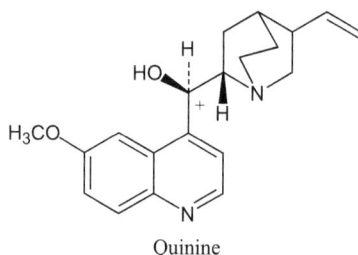

Quinine

Fig. (2). Chemical structure of Quinine.

Isolation

Cinchona coarse powder is mixed with 30% of its weight with calcium hydroxide and 5% NaOH solution and allowed to stand for a few hours to release the free alkaloid. The mass is then extracted with benzene for 6 hours in the Soxhlet apparatus. The benzene extract is shaken with 5% H_2SO_4 to convert the alkaloid bases into water-soluble salts. The pH of the aqueous acid extract is adjusted to 6.5 with dil. NaOH. The extract is cooled and allowed to stand for some time. Neutral quinine sulfate crystals are isolated from cinchonine and cinchonidine by repeated crystallization for hot water.

5.4. Solasodine

Solasodine (Fig. **3**) is isolated from dried berries of *Solanum khasianum* and *S. dulcamara* (Solanaceae). The berries contain about 3% of steroidal glycoalkaloid called solasodine. Mucilage surrounding part of the seeds contains the highest amount of alkaloid. Immature and over-ripe fruits contain negligible content of alkaloid, while it is at the maximum when fruits change color from green to yellow. Solasodine is used as a precursor for steroidal synthesis. Like Diosgenin, it is first converted to 16-dehydro-pregnenelone acetate. The latter is a precursor for steroids, like corticosteroids, pregnane, androstanes and 19-Nor steroids. All of these are useful as sex hormones, oral contraceptives.

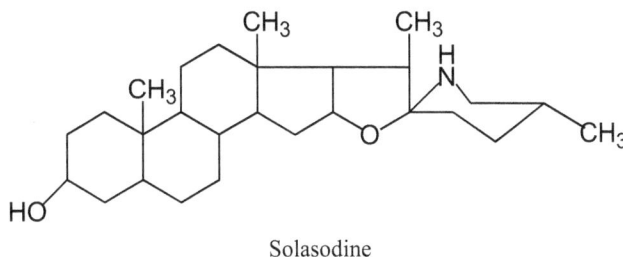

Solasodine

Fig. (3). Chemical structure of Solasodine.

Isolation

The berries are powdered and the oil is removed by defatting. The defatted material is extracted with ethanol. The concentrated extract is treated with conc. HCl, and 6 hours of reflux. After that, ammonia is applied to basify the extract and refluxed again for 1 hour. It is filtered and the residue of chloroform is washed dried and dissolved. This mixture is filtered and solasodine in the form of residue is obtained by evaporating the solvent.

5.5. Caffeine

Caffeine (1,3,7-trimethylxanthine) is a purine alkaloid obtained from leaves and leaf buds of *Thea sinensis (Camellia thea)* (Theaceae) and dried ripe seed of *Coffea arabica* Linn. or *C. lberica* Hiern (Rubiaceae). Beverages such as tea and coffee owe their stimulant properties because of caffeine (Fig. **4**).

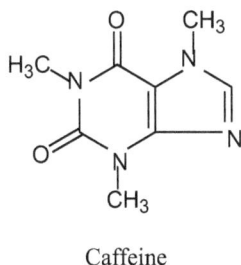

Caffeine

Fig. (4). Chemical structure of Caffeine.

Isolation

1. Approximately 50 g of tea leaves or roasted coffee powder is extracted with 300 ml water in a beaker for 20 minutes containing $NaHCO_3$ (10 g).
2. The solution is filtered while it is hot, the filtrate is neutralized with 10% H_2SO_4 solution.
3. The filtrate is again extracted with dichloromethane in separating funnel.
4. The organic layer is combined and the solvent is evaporated.

5. Crude caffeine is purified by dissolving the residue in a minimum volume of the acetone and kept for some time, it gets the silky needles shaped crystals of caffeine.

5.6. Starch

Starch consists of polysaccharide granules obtained from the grains of Maize (*Zea mays* Linn.), Rice (*Oryza sativa* Linn.) or Wheat (*Triticum aestivum* Linn.) belonging to the family Gramineae or from the tubers of Potato (*Solanum tuberosum* Linn.) belonging to family Solanaceae.

Starch contains chemically different polysaccharides: amylose (β-amylose) and amylopectin (α-amylose), about 80%. Amylose is water-soluble and amylopectin is water-insoluble, but swells in water and is responsible for the gelatinizing property of the starch. Amylose gives blue color with iodine, while amylopectin yields bluish-black coloration with iodine. Starch finds extensive use in dusting powders, in which its absorbent properties are important. In mucilage form, it is used as a skin emollient, as a basis for some enemas and as an antidote in the treatment of iodine poisoning. Starch is also used as a tablet disintegrant. Starch is used as nutritive, demulcent, protective and as an absorbent. Starch is also used as a starting material for the commercial preparation of liquid glucose, dextrose, and dextrin.

Isolation of starch from potatoes.

1. Wash the potatoes thoroughly with water to remove adhering soil and earthy matter.
2. Chop the potatoes to small pieces and make them into a fine slurry with water in a blender.
3. Pass the slurry through a muslin cloth to remove the cell debris and other impurities.
4. Again pass the slurry through metallic sieves to effectively remove the cell debris and other impurities.
5. Allow the milky layer to settle down and decant the supernatant liquid.
6. Wash the sediments (containing starch), 2-3 times with distilled water with constant stirring.
7. Centrifuge the milky liquid and dry the pellet of starch in an oven at temperature (35-40°C) and grind it to powder. Temperature more than 60°C will gelatinize the starch.

5.7. Menthol

Menthol (Fig. **5**) is found in mentha oil obtained from *Mentha arvensis* (Labiatae). Menthol is also present in the oil of peppermint (*Mentha piperita,* Labiatae) to the extent of about 80%. Menthol is monoterpene alcohol obtained in levorotatory form *i.e.* (-) menthol, which is assigned the (1R,2S,5R) configuration. Synthetic menthol is racemic (±) mixture. Pure (-)-menthol has four crystal forms, of which the most stable is the α-form, the familiar broad needles. It is used for the treatment of headaches, muscle cramps and sprains. It also a component of formulation used in cough medicines, lip balms and gargles.

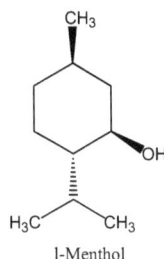

l-Menthol

Fig. (5). Chemical structure of l-Menthol.

Isolation

1. Mentha oil, the basic raw material for menthol is obtained by steam distillation of the *Mentha arvensis* crop.
2. The mentha oil obtained is subjected to a series of fractional chilling to give needle-shaped l-menthol crystals.
3. The crystals of menthol are further purified by elaborating crystallization technique to get bold crystals of high purity.

5.8. Artemisinin

Artemisinin (Fig. **6**) is a quadricyclic sesquiterpene lactone isolated from *Artemisia annua* (Asteraceae). Artemisinin is discovered by Tu Youyou in 1972 in China, for this discovery she received a Nobel prize in 2015. World Health Organization (WHO) recommends the toxin-free, artemisinin-based combination therapy (ACT) as the most effective against drug-resistant malaria.

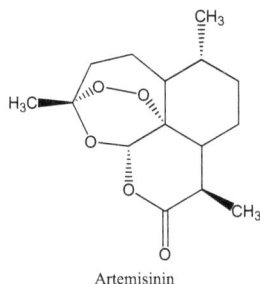

Artemisinin

Fig. (6). Chemical structure of Artemisinin.

Isolation

About 100 g of coarse powder *A. annua* is macerated using ethanol (250 ml) for 24 hrs. The solution is filtered and the filtrate is partitioned with 100 ml of hexane. Further, 100 ml of distilled water was added to the ethanol extract and partitioned again using 100 ml of ethyl acetate (thrice). Each extract is combined and concentrated using a rotavapor at a temperature of 40 °C. The extract is subjected to column chromatography using a mixture of ethyl acetate-hexane with increasing polarity as eluents that leads to isolation of artemisinin.

5.9. Reserpine

Reserpine (Fig. **7**) is isolated from the root and rhizome of *Rauwolfia serpentiana* (Apocynaceae). Reserpine is an indole alkaloid possessing indole as a part of its structure. The compound has two nitrogen atoms, one is present in the indole nucleus and the other is two carbons apart from the β-position of the indole ring. Reserpine is used for the treatment of hypertension.

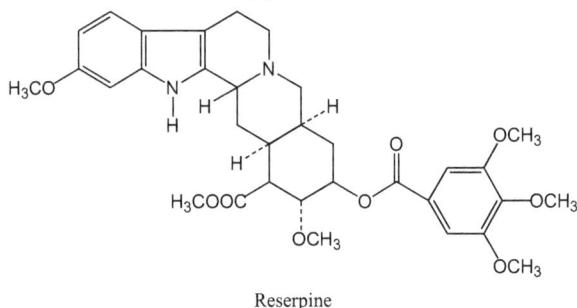

Reserpine

Fig. (7). Chemical structure of Reserpine.

Isolation

About 250 g of *Rauwolfia* root powder with 2.5 L of the ether-benzene-ethanol mixture is shaken for 15 minutes and filtered. Add aqueous ammonium hydroxide to the filtrate, and continued shaking for 48 hours and then filter. Combine the extracts and concentrate under vacuum using rota evaporator and finally dried over sodium sulfate. The residue, dissolved in 200 ml of benzene, was chromatographed on 75 g of neutral alumina using ether-chloroform as eluents. The pooled ether-chloroform eluates after crystallization from methanol yielded 117 mg of reserpine with m.p. 262-263 °C.

5.10. Digitoxin

Digitoxin (Fig. **8**) occurs in the leaves of *Digitalis purpurea* and *D. lanata* of family Scrophulariaceae along with other cardiac glycosides like gitoxin, gitaloxin, lanatosides *etc.*

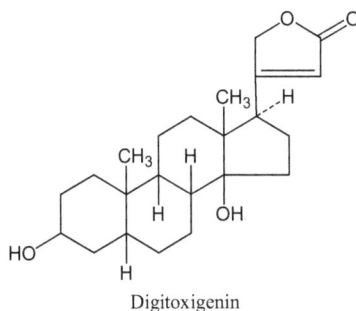

Digitoxigenin

Fig. (8). Chemical structure of Digitoxigenin.

Digitoxin is a cardiac glycoside, the aglycone moiety is called digitoxigenin, which is C_{23} cardenolide having α,β-unsaturated five-membered lactone ring attached at 17-β position. The glycone part is three digitoxose sugar which is attached linearly and form glycosidic bond at C-3 of aglycone part. It is used for the treatment of congestive heart failure. Digitalis blocks the sodium-potassium ATPase pump of the cardiac muscles so that intra-cellular concentration of sodium is increased. This leads to an increase in calcium ions released from sarcolemma, and proteins actin and myosin enhanced which exhibited more forceful contractions of myocardium.

Isolation

The powdered drug is macerated for 4-5 hours at 45 °C with water and the aqueous extract is collected. The marc is macerated with 20% methanol for 24 hr and the methanolic extract is collected. The aqueous and methanolic extracts are mixed with NaOH and are made alkaline to induce hydrolysis. This is then removed and evaporated with chloroform to dryness. The residue is subjected to column chromatography using eluents as ethyl acetate and methanol.

6. CONCLUDING REMARKS

The role of natural products in drug discovery and development is paramount. Since ancient times natural products are the only remedies available to cure human ailments. Due to recent development in extraction and isolation techniques, drug discovery from natural resources becomes fast and easy. In the meantime, new automated and fast technology for the extraction and separation of natural products has been developed. Regarding the classical method of extraction, percolation is the most important extraction method and is commonly employed for the preparation of homeopathic formulations. Modern extraction techniques such as UAE, MAE, PLE, SFE and enzyme assisted extraction methods are also applied for the extraction of bioactive phytochemicals in sample preparation for further quantitative analysis or for isolation and structural elucidation of phytochemicals in the drug discovery and development.

CONSENT FOR PUBLICATION

Not applicable.

CONFLICT OF INTEREST

The author(s) confirms that there is no conflict of interest.

ACKNOWLEDGEMENTS

Declared none.

REFERENCES

[1]   Mukherji PK. Quality control on herbal drugs. New Delhi: Eastern Publishers (Business Horizons Ltd.) 2002; p. 816.

[2]   Smith RM. Before the injection--modern methods of sample preparation for separation techniques. J Chromatogr A 2003; 1000(1-2): 3-27.
[http://dx.doi.org/10.1016/S0021-9673(03)00511-9] [PMID: 12877164]

[3]   Sasidharan S, Chen Y, Saravanan D, Sundram KM, Yoga Latha L. Extraction, isolation and characterization of bioactive compounds from plants' extracts. Afr J Tradit Complement Altern Med 2011; 8(1): 1-10.
[PMID: 22238476]

[4]   Zhang QW, Lin LG, Ye WC. Techniques for extraction and isolation of natural products: a comprehensive review. Chin Med 2018; 13(20): 20.
[http://dx.doi.org/10.1186/s13020-018-0177-x] [PMID: 29692864]

[5]   Ahamad J, Amin S, Mir SR. Optimization of ultrasound-assisted extraction of charantin from

Momordica charantia fruits using response surface methodology. J Pharm Bioallied Sci 2015; 7(4): 304-7.
[http://dx.doi.org/10.4103/0975-7406.168032] [PMID: 26681889]

[6] Harborne JB. Phytochemical methods-A guide to modern technique of plant analysis. 3rd ed. London: Chapman and Hall 1998; pp. 109-45.

[7] Ahamad J, Amin S, Mir SR. Response surface methodology for optimization of ultrasound assisted extraction of swertiamarin from *Enicostema littorale* Blume. Curr Bioact Compd 2016; 12: 87-92.
[http://dx.doi.org/10.2174/1573407212021605042222203]

[8] Ćujić N, Šavikin K, Janković T, Pljevljakušić D, Zdunić G, Ibrić S. Optimization of polyphenols extraction from dried chokeberry using maceration as traditional technique. Food Chem 2016; 194: 135-42.
[http://dx.doi.org/10.1016/j.foodchem.2015.08.008] [PMID: 26471536]

[9] Albuquerque BR, Prieto MA, Barreiro MF, *et al.* Catechin-based extract optimization obtained from *Arbutus unedo* L. fruits using maceration/ microwave/ ultrasound extraction techniques. Ind Crops Prod 2017; 95: 404-15.
[http://dx.doi.org/10.1016/j.indcrop.2016.10.050]

[10] Li SL, Lai SF, Song JZ, *et al.* Decocting-induced chemical transformations and global quality of Du-Shen-Tang, the decoction of ginseng evaluated by UPLC-Q-TOF-MS/MS based chemical profiling approach. J Pharm Biomed Anal 2010; 53(4): 946-57.
[http://dx.doi.org/10.1016/j.jpba.2010.07.001] [PMID: 20667431]

[11] Zhang WL, Chen JP, Lam KYC, *et al.* Hydrolysis of glycosidic favonoids during the preparation of Danggui Buxue Tang: an outcome of moderate boiling of Chinese herbal mixture. Evid Based Complement Altern Med 2014; p. 608721.

[12] Zhang H, Wang W, Fu ZM, Han CC, Song Y. Study on comparison of extracting fucoxanthin from *Undaria pinnatifda* with percolation extraction and refluxing methods. Zhongguo Shipin Tianjiaji 2014; 9: 91-5.

[13] Kongkiatpaiboon S, Gritsanapan W. Optimized extraction for high yield of insecticidal didehydrostemofoline alkaloid in *Stemona collinsiae* root extracts. Ind Crops Prod 2013; 41: 371-4.
[http://dx.doi.org/10.1016/j.indcrop.2012.04.047]

[14] Zhang L. Comparison of extraction effect of active ingredients in traditional Chinese medicine compound preparation with two different methods. Heilongjiang Xumu Shouyi 2013; 9: 132-3.

[15] Wei Q, Yang GW, Wang XJ, Hu XX, Chen L. The study on optimization of Soxhlet extraction process for ursolic acid from *Cynomorium*. Shipin Yanjiu Yu Kaifa 2013; 34(7): 85-8.

[16] Chin FS, Chong KP, Markus A, Wong NK. Tea polyphenols and alkaloids content using Soxhlet and direct extraction methods. World J Agric Sci 2013; 9(3): 266-70.

[17] Yahya A, Yunus RM. Influence of sample preparation and extraction time on chemical composition of steam distillation derived patchouli oil. Proc Eng 2013; 53: 1-6.
[http://dx.doi.org/10.1016/j.proeng.2013.02.001]

[18] Hamad KJ, Al-Shaheen SJA, Kaskoos RA, Javed A, Jameel M, Mir SR. Essential oil composition and antioxidant activity of *Lavandula angustifolia* from Iraq. Int Res J Pharm 2013; 4(4): 117-20.

[19] Naquvi KJ, Ahamad J, Ali M, Ansari SH, Salma A. Analysis of essential oil of *Origanum vulgare* Linn by GC and GC-MS. J Glob Trends Pharm Sci 2018; 9(3): 5786-91.

[20] Ahamad J, Uthirapathy S, Ameen MSM, Anwer ET. Essential oil composition and antidiabetic, anticancer activity of Rosmarinus officinalis L leaves from Erbil. Iraq: J Essent Oil Bearing Plants 2019.
[http://dx.doi.org/10.1080/0972060X.2019.1689179]

[21] Mason TJ, Paniwnyk L, Lorimer JP. The uses of ultrasound in food technology. Ultrason Sonochem

1996; 3(3): 253-60.
[http://dx.doi.org/10.1016/S1350-4177(96)00034-X]

[22]   Kamaljit V, Raymond M, Lloyd S, Darren B. Applications and opportunities for ultrasound assisted extraction in the food industry- A review. Innov Food Sci Emerg Technol 2008; 9: 161-9.
[http://dx.doi.org/10.1016/j.ifset.2007.04.014]

[23]   Pan G, Yu G, Zhu C, Qiao J. Optimization of ultrasound-assisted extraction (UAE) of flavonoids compounds (FC) from hawthorn seed (HS). Ultrason Sonochem 2012; 19(3): 486-90.
[http://dx.doi.org/10.1016/j.ultsonch.2011.11.006] [PMID: 22142939]

[24]   Rostagno MA, Palma M, Barroso CG. Ultrasound-assisted extraction of soy isoflavones. J Chromatogr A 2003; 1012(2): 119-28.
[http://dx.doi.org/10.1016/S0021-9673(03)01184-1] [PMID: 14521308]

[25]   Yang Y, Zhang F. Ultrasound-assisted extraction of rutin and quercetin from *Euonymus alatus* (Thunb.) Sieb. Ultrason Sonochem 2008; 15(4): 308-13.
[http://dx.doi.org/10.1016/j.ultsonch.2007.05.001] [PMID: 17606398]

[26]   Yang L, Wang H, Zu Y, *et al.* Ultrasound-assisted extraction of the three terpenoid indole alkaloids vindoline, catharanthine and vinblastine from *Catharanthus roseus* using ionic liquid aqueous solutions. Chem Eng J 2011; 172(2-3): 705-12.
[http://dx.doi.org/10.1016/j.cej.2011.06.039]

[27]   Ghafoor K, Choi YH, Jeon JY, Jo IH. Optimization of ultrasound-assisted extraction of phenolic compounds, antioxidants, and anthocyanins from grape (*Vitis vinifera*) seeds. J Agric Food Chem 2009; 57(11): 4988-94.
[http://dx.doi.org/10.1021/jf9001439] [PMID: 19405527]

[28]   Ghafoor K, Hui T, Choi YH. Optimization of ultrasound-assisted extraction of total anthocyanins from grape peel. J Food Biochem 2011; 35: 735-46.
[http://dx.doi.org/10.1111/j.1745-4514.2010.00413.x]

[29]   Zu G, Zhang R, Yang L, *et al.* Ultrasound-assisted extraction of carnosic acid and rosmarinic acid using ionic liquid solution from *Rosmarinus officinalis*. Int J Mol Sci 2012; 13(9): 11027-43.
[http://dx.doi.org/10.3390/ijms130911027] [PMID: 23109836]

[30]   Melecchi MI, Péres VF, Dariva C, *et al.* Optimization of the sonication extraction method of *Hibiscus tiliaceus* L. flowers. Ultrason Sonochem 2006; 13(3): 242-50.
[http://dx.doi.org/10.1016/j.ultsonch.2005.02.003] [PMID: 15993639]

[31]   Hu T, Guo YY, Zhou QF, *et al.* Optimization of ultrasonic-assisted extraction of total saponins from *Eclipta prostrasta* L. using response surface methodology. J Food Sci 2012; 77(9): C975-82.
[http://dx.doi.org/10.1111/j.1750-3841.2012.02869.x] [PMID: 22900526]

[32]   Chen W, Wang WP, Zhang HS, Huang Q. Optimization of ultrasonic-assisted extraction of water-soluble polysaccharides from *Boletus edulis* mycelia using response surface methodology. Carbohydr Polym 2012; 87(1): 614-9.
[http://dx.doi.org/10.1016/j.carbpol.2011.08.029]

[33]   Ahamad J, Amin S, Mir SR. Optimization of Ultrasonic-Assisted Extraction of Gymnemic Acid from *Gymnema sylvestre* leaves using Response Surface Methodology. Anal Chem Lett 2014; 4(2): 104-12.
[http://dx.doi.org/10.1080/22297928.2014.905754]

[34]   Letellier M, Budzinski H. Microwave assisted extraction of organic compounds. Analysis 1999; 27(3): 259-70.

[35]   Pan X, Niu G, Liu H. Microwave-assisted extraction of tea polyphenols and tea caffeine from green tea leaves. Chem Eng Process 2003; 42(2): 129-33.
[http://dx.doi.org/10.1016/S0255-2701(02)00037-5]

[36]   Shu YY, Ko MY, Chang YS. Microwave-assisted extraction of ginsenosides from ginseng root. Microchem J 2003; 74(2): 131-9.

[http://dx.doi.org/10.1016/S0026-265X(02)00180-7]

[37]   Dhobi M, Mandal V, Hemalatha S. Optimization of microwave assisted extraction of bioactive flavolignin-silybinin. J Chem Metrol 2009; 3(1): 13-23.

[38]   Asghari J, Ondruschka B, Mazaheritehrani M. Extraction of bioactive chemical compounds from the medicinal Asian plants by microwave irradiation. J Med Plants Res 2011; 5(4): 495-506.

[39]   Chiremba C, Rooney LW, Beta T. Microwave-assisted extraction of bound phenolic acids in bran and flour fractions from sorghum and maize cultivars varying in hardness. J Agric Food Chem 2012; 60(18): 4735-42.
[http://dx.doi.org/10.1021/jf300279t] [PMID: 22500656]

[40]   Hui T, Ghafoor K, Choi YH. Optimization of microwave-assisted extraction of active components from Chinese quince using response surface methodology. J Korean Soc Appl Biol Chem 2009; 52(6): 694-701.
[http://dx.doi.org/10.3839/jksabc.2009.115]

[41]   Ibanez E, Herrero M, Mendiola JA, Castro-Puyana M. Extraction and characterization of bioactive compounds with health benefits from marine resources: macro and micro algae, cyanobacteria, and invertebrates.Marine bioactive compounds: sources, characterization and applications. Springer 2012; pp. 55-98.
[http://dx.doi.org/10.1007/978-1-4614-1247-2_2]

[42]   Rostagno MA, Palma M, Barroso CG. Pressurized liquid extraction of isoflavones from soybeans. Anal Chim Acta 2004; 522(2): 169-77.
[http://dx.doi.org/10.1016/j.aca.2004.05.078]

[43]   Shen J, Shao X. A comparison of accelerated solvent extraction, Soxhlet extraction, and ultrasonic-assisted extraction for analysis of terpenoids and sterols in tobacco. Anal Bioanal Chem 2005; 383(6): 1003-8.
[http://dx.doi.org/10.1007/s00216-005-0078-6] [PMID: 16231136]

[44]   Luthria DL. Influence of experimental conditions on the extraction of phenolic compounds from parsley (*Petroselinum crispum*) flakes using a pressurized liquid extractor. Food Chem 2008; 107(2): 745-52.
[http://dx.doi.org/10.1016/j.foodchem.2007.08.074]

[45]   Mroczek T, Mazurek J. Pressurized liquid extraction and anticholinesterase activity-based thin-layer chromatography with bioautography of Amaryllidaceae alkaloids. Anal Chim Acta 2009; 633(2): 188-96.
[http://dx.doi.org/10.1016/j.aca.2008.11.053] [PMID: 19166722]

[46]   Erdogan S, Ates B, Durmaz G, Yilmaz I, Seckin T. Pressurized liquid extraction of phenolic compounds from *Anatolia propolis* and their radical scavenging capacities. Food Chem Toxicol 2011; 49(7): 1592-7.
[http://dx.doi.org/10.1016/j.fct.2011.04.006] [PMID: 21530603]

[47]   Sihvonen M, Jarvenpaa E, Hietaniemi V, Huopalahti R. Advances in supercritical carbon dioxide technologies. Trends Food Sci Technol 1999; 10(6-7): 217-22.
[http://dx.doi.org/10.1016/S0924-2244(99)00049-7]

[48]   Saldaña MDA, Mohamed RS, Baer MG, Mazzafera P. Extraction of purine alkaloids from maté (*Ilex paraguariensis*) using supercritical $CO_{(2)}$. J Agric Food Chem 1999; 47(9): 3804-8.
[http://dx.doi.org/10.1021/jf981369z] [PMID: 10552725]

[49]   Giannuzzo AN, Boggetti HJ, Nazareno MA, Mishima HT. Supercritical fluid extraction of naringin from the peel of Citrus paradisi. Phytochem Anal 2003; 14(4): 221-3.
[http://dx.doi.org/10.1002/pca.706] [PMID: 12892417]

[50]   Ashraf-Khorassani M, Taylor LT. Sequential fractionation of grape seeds into oils, polyphenols, and procyanidins *via* a single system employing CO_2-based fluids. J Agric Food Chem 2004; 52(9): 2440-

4.
[http://dx.doi.org/10.1021/jf030510n] [PMID: 15113138]

[51]   Verma A, Hartonen K, Riekkola ML. Optimisation of supercritical fluid extraction of indole alkaloids from *Catharanthus roseus* using experimental design methodology--comparison with other extraction techniques. Phytochem Anal 2008; 19(1): 52-63.
[http://dx.doi.org/10.1002/pca.1015] [PMID: 17654538]

[52]   Chen H, Zhou X, Zhang J. Optimization of enzyme assisted extraction of polysaccharides from *Astragalus membranaceus.* Carbohydr Polym 2014; 111: 567-75.
[http://dx.doi.org/10.1016/j.carbpol.2014.05.033] [PMID: 25037388]

[53]   Strati IF, Gogou E, Oreopoulou V. Enzyme and high pressure assisted extraction of carotenoids from tomato waste. Food Bioprod Process 2015; 94: 668-74.
[http://dx.doi.org/10.1016/j.fbp.2014.09.012]

[54]   Liu T, Sui X, Li L, *et al.* Application of ionic liquids based enzyme-assisted extraction of chlorogenic acid from *Eucommia ulmoides* leaves. Anal Chim Acta 2016; 903: 91-9.
[http://dx.doi.org/10.1016/j.aca.2015.11.029] [PMID: 26709302]

CHAPTER 4

Isolation and Purification of Bioactive Phytochemicals

Kamran Javed Naquvi[1,*], **Javed Ahamad**[2], **Raad A Kaskoos**[3], **Naila Hasan Ali Alkefai**[4], **Afrin Salma**[5] and **Showkat R. Mir**[6]

[1] *Department of Pharmacognosy & Phytochemistry, Faculty of Pharmaceutical Sciences, Rama University, Rama City, Mandhana, Kanpur (Uttar Pradesh) - 209 217, India*

[2] *Department of Pharmacognosy, Faculty of Pharmacy, Tishk International University, Erbil, Kurdistan Region, Iraq*

[3] *Faculty of Pharmacy, Howler Medical University, Kurdistan Region, Iraq*

[4] *Department of Pharmacognosy, Faculty of Pharmacy, University of Hafer Albatin, Hafer Albatin, KSA*

[5] *Department of Pharmaceutical Chemistry, Translum Institute of Pharmaceutical Education and Research, Meerut (UP), India*

[6] *Department of Pharmacognosy, School of Pharmaceutical Education and Research, Jamia Hamdard, New Delhi, India*

Abstract: Various forms of natural products such as plant extracts, pure phytochemicals and herbal formulations containing natural products offer tremendous opportunities for new drug discoveries and the credit goes to its chemical diversity. Since time immemorial medicinal plants in its various forms and have been used to treat chronic diseases such as malaria, tuberculosis, cardiovascular diseases, *etc.* Recently along with the crude form of medicinal plants and their isolated active principles are also being used to cure several maladies. Isolation of bioactive constituents from the medicinal plants has always been a challenge because of the complexities involved in separation process, but the recent technological advancement in this field has facilitated the isolation process of chemical constituents from the plants. This book chapter offers a comprehensive review on the procedural techniques and application of classical column chromatography, prep-TLC, modern isolation and purification techniques such as flash chromatography, prep-HPLC, prep-GC, counter current chromatography, *etc.*

Keywords: Column Chromatography, Counter-Current Chromatography, Flash Chromatography, Isolation, Natural Products, Phytochemicals, Preparative-GC, Preparative-HPLC, Preparative-TLC, Purification.

* **Corresponding author Dr. Kamran Javed Naquvi:** Department of Pharmacognosy & Phytochemistry, Faculty of Pharmaceutical Sciences, Rama University, Rama City, Mandhana, Kanpur (Uttar Pradesh) - 209 217, India; E-mail: kjnaquvi@gmail.com

Javed Ahmad and Javed Ahamad (Ed.)

1. INTRODUCTION

Medicinal plants have been reported to be repository of various types of bioactive compounds, which possessing tremendous therapeutic properties. The use of plants as a therapeutic agent over a very long time period has been established. The magnificent and diverse plant kingdom is well known for its medicinal values. Herbal therapies across the globe for various diseases are largely dependent on the therapeutic potential of medicinal plants [1]. Plants are being used for medicinal purposes long before the prehistoric era. Since ancient times scholars from Egypt, India, China and Arabian countries compiled and utilized herbs as medicinal agents and fulfilled their basic health care needs from these medicinal herbs. Herbal therapies have been considered as the safest one because of their minimal or no side effect characteristics. As these remedies do align with the nature and hence offer the biggest advantage. One of the facts relating to herbal treatments is that it is independent of any age group and the sexes. Natural flora is considered as one of the richest and biodiverse resource of active ingredients, which can be used for pharmacopeial, non-pharmacopeial or synthetic drug development. Moreover, some plants also possess nutritional values along with their therapeutic potential and hence they are the most recommended ones in the therapeutic domain [2].

Drug discovery and development is a complex, time consuming and very expensive process. Drug discovery process involves the identification of new chemical entities (NCES), which should possess the desired pharmacokinetic and pharmacodynamic properties. The NCES are generally obtained through isolation from natural resources or through chemical syntheses. In the pre genomic era and when there was no high throughput screening (HTS), more than 80% of drug substances were plant based or were the derivatives of plant based medicines [3, 4]. Newman and Cragg, reported that total 1562 new drugs were approved during 1981 to 2014, out of which natural products (4%; N), derivatives of natural products (21%, ND), synthetic compounds with natural product-derived pharmacophores (10%; S*/NM), and synthetic drug with NP pharmacophore (11%; S/NM). From the above report it is clear that about 51% of the drugs discovered come directly or indirectly from natural products [5].

WHO estimated about 20,000 plants having medicinal values exist in 91 countries including 12 mega biodiverse countries. Natural products isolated from plants offer unparalleled source of chemical diversity for the discovery of biologically active scaffolds [6]. The critical steps for revelation of the biologically active compounds from plant resources are extraction, isolation, characterization and pharmacological screening of bioactive compounds followed by toxicological and clinical evaluation. Considering the fact that plant extract happened to possess a combination of various types of bioactive compounds or the plant constituents with different polarities, their separation still poses a great challenge for the process of identification and characterization of bioactive compounds [7].

Isolation of single constituents from plant generally involves separation of components from its mixture (extract). The separated single constituents might contain impurities which are further separated by several purification processes. Purification refers to the process of separating or extracting the target compound from other (possibly structurally related) compounds or contaminants. Generally chromatographic methods are employed for separation and purification of bioactive chemicals from plants. For isolation of single component mostly column chromatography, prep-TLC, counter-current chromatography is applied and for purification, prep-HPLC, MPLC is used [8 - 10]. Isolation and purification of the bioactive phytochemicals from medicinal plants have always posed the problems associated with their chemical complexities. Recent technological advancements related to isolation and separation techniques have made the process quite easier than before [11]. For the isolation and purification purpose, various solvents with differential polarities either individually or in combination are used. Bioactive guided fractionation and isolation of phytochemicals are now practiced widely. Preparative thin layer chromatography (prep-TLC) and column chromatography are the oldest chromatographic methods applied for isolation and purification of bioactive phytochemicals from plant sources. These traditional methods are still the first choice due to their convenience with respect to the economic feasibility and availability in various stationary phases [12]. Recent advancement in isolation and purification techniques leads to develop more sophisticated instruments such as preparative high pressured liquid chromatography (prep-HPLC), countercurrent chromatography (CCC), and medium pressure liquid chromatography (MPLC) which expedites the process of isolation and purification of bioactive compounds [13]. In this book chapter we have compiled a comprehensive overlook about isolation and purification techniques such as prep-TLC, prep-HPLC, CCC, MPLC and preparative gas chromatography (prep-GC).

2. TECHNIQUES OF NATURAL PRODUCT ISOLATION

2.1. Counter-Current Chromatography (CCC)

Natural product extracts contain mixtures of highly complex compounds; because of this reason the purification process becomes a highly challenging task. Purification protocols sometimes take months or years, as it involves isolation of a single active molecule from the hundreds of compounds that can be present in the complex mixture form in an extract. Thus it is critical for a phytochemist to develop a wide range of isolation and purification techniques [14]. Counter-current chromatography (CCC) is a sophisticated, fast, reliable and reproducible technique emerged for isolation and purification of bioactive phytochemicals. In CCC the separation of chemical compounds based on type of liquid partition chromatography by using a separation column devoid of solid matrix. CCC provides advantages over excessive loss and deactivation of phytochemicals [11].

In a holistic way, countercurrent chromatography is based on chromatography concepts in which one is stationary and the other is mobile without any substantial support [15, 16]. The counter-current chromatography comprises a chamber connected to a number of hollow tubes that contain liquid stationary and mobile phases. The plant sample is injected with solvent and mobile phase is pumped through a series of hollow tubes. The separation of components occurs due to difference in solubility of the two phases because of applied dynamic mixing and settling action. In this technique wide range of mobile phase are used for obtaining proper separation [17, 18].

There are various types of countercurrent chromatography like dual flow countercurrent chromatography (DFCCC) featuring a true countercurrent process where the biphasic system flows past each other and leave at opposite ends of the column [19]. The concept of chromatography can be understood as, the one liquid acts as the stationary phase by retaining in the column while the other one being pumped out can be considered as the mobile phase. There are two ways by which the stationary phase is returned in the column: hydrostatic centrifugal force and hydrodynamic centrifugal force. In the hydrostatic method the column is rotated about the central axis [20, 21] and it is commonly known as centrifugal partition chromatography (CPC) [22]. Instruments based on hydrodynamic centrifugation commonly called as high speed or high performance counter current chromatography (HSCCC), and it applies Archimedes Force to retain stationary phase in column [23].

Droplet countercurrent chromatography was introduced in 1970 [20]. This technique is depending on gravitational force for the movement of mobile phase through the stationary phase. The mobile phase travels through long hollow tubes connected to chamber where separation occurs. In descending mode of separation, mobile phase droplets pass through columns of lightest stationary phase with the help of gravitational force [24]. In ascending mode, the mobile phase is selected to possess lesser density than the stationary phase so that it can run upward. The eluent from one column is allowed to pass through another column leading to achieve more theoretical plates. The mobile phase in this method is pumped at such a rate which allows the droplets to be formed and maximize the mass transfer of a compound between the two phases.

Here the separation is based on the relative solubility of the compounds in the two phases and the ratio of their solubility in different phases is called the partition coefficient. The biphasic solvent system should be designed in such a way that it performs appropriately in the DCCC column. The densities of the two phases should also be sufficiency varying in such a way that both should facilitate the movement of each other to pass through in a column. Many DCCC solvent systems consist of chloroform and water. Solvent systems consisting of n-butanol, water and a modifier for example acetic acid, pyridine or *n*-propanol have achieved success to some extent in DCCC system [25]. Slow flow rates and poor mixing was the largest setback for most binary solvent systems. These techniques have been used for isolation of the wide variety of chemical compounds from plant extracts, some examples are illustrated in Table **1**.

Table 1. Examples of phytochemicals isolated by counter-current chromatography.

Phytochemicals	Source Plants	Solvent System	Techniques	References
Saponins (triterpenoid glycosides)	*Hedera helix* berries	$CHCl_3$,-MeOH-H_2O (5:6:4)	DCCC	[25]
Sarsapogenin-O-β-D-xylopy-ranosyl-(1 → 2) β-D-galacto-pyranoside, sarsapogenin-O-β-D-glucopyranosyl (1 → 2)-β-D-galactopyranoside	*Cornus florida* L.	$CHCl_3$-MeOH-H_2O (7:13:8)	DCCC	[26]
Parthenolide and related sesquiterpene lactones	Asteraceae plants	Benzene - chloroform - methanol -water; chloroform-trichloroethylene - acetonitrile - methanol - water	DCCC	[27]
Coclaurine	*Zizyphus jujuba*	C_6H_6: $CHCl_3$:MeOH: H_2O (5:5:7:2)	DCCC	[28]
Xanthones	*Gentianas trictiflora*	$CHCl_3$/MeOH/H_2O (65: 35: 20)	DCCC	[25]
Iridoid glycusides	*Ajuga pyramidalis*	$CHCl_3$/MeOH/H_2O (43:37:20)	DCCC	[25]
β-Carotene, lutein, violaxanthin and neoxanthin	*Petroselinum crispum*	Petroleum spirit (b.p. 40–60°C): acetonitrile: methanol (50:10:40)	DCCC	[29]
Flavonoid glycosides	Several plant species	*n*-BuOH-AcOH-H_2O (4:1:5)	DCCC	[25]
Nor-seco-triterpene and penta-cyclic triterpenoids like belle-ricagenin B, bellericaside B and arjunglucoside I, 28-*nor*-17, 22-*seco*-2α, 3β, 19, 22, 23-pentahydroxy-Δ12-oleanane	*Qualea parviflora*	$CHCl_3$/MeOH/H_2O (43:37:20, v/v)	DCCC	[30]

(Table 1) cont.....

Phytochemicals	Source Plants	Solvent System	Techniques	References
Procyanidin B1-B4; Procyanidin B2-3'-*O*-gallate, Procyanidin C1	Grape seeds	*n*-hexane - ethyl acetate - water (1:50:50, v/v/v)	HSCCC	[31]
Polymeric proanthocyanidins	Grape seeds	*n*-hexane - ethyl acetate - water (1:80:80, v/v/v)	HSCCC	[32]
Gallic acid, methyl gallate, and epigallocatechin-3-gallate	Persimmon	*n*-hexane - ethyl acetate - water (3:17:20, v/v/v) and ethyl acetate-methanol-water (50:1:50, v/v/v)	HSCCC	[33]

2.2. Column Chromatography (CC)

This is a classic example of liquid solid chromatography in which the mobile phase passes through the finely divided stationary phase, filled in a glass column. Here the driving force for movement of mobile phase is the gravitational force only. This is considered as one of the most common and acceptable technique, because of the availability of wide range of solvents and various adsorbents. Column chromatography can be used on scales for micrograms up to kilograms. The relatively low-cost and controllability of the stationary phase can be regarded as the main advantage with this technique [34]. Column chromatography can be regarded as one of the most commonly used technique for separation of compounds in pharmacy laboratory as well as in industries. Although with the advent of newer, expensive and sophisticated chromatographic techniques as medium pressure liquid chromatography and counter-current chromatography; column chromatography is losing its space in advanced research laboratories [35]. Column chromatography is generally works on two principals: adsorption column chromatography (which mixture components are adsorbed on adsorbent surfaces) and partition column chromatography (the stationary as well as the mobile phases are in liquid stage). Adsorption column chromatography is of mainly normal-phase chromatography and reverse phase chromatography. In normal-phase chromatography, the stationary phase is polar such silica gel and mobile phase ranges from non-polar to medium polar such as petroleum ether, chloroform, ethyl acetate, *etc*. In reverse phase column chromatography, the stationary phases are mostly non-polar such as C18 and C8 chain bonded with silica and mobile phases are polar such as acetonitrile methanol, water, *etc*. [34]. Generally dry and wet methods are commonly used for the preparation of the column. In the first method, column is gradually filled with the finely divided stationary powder and tapped occasionally followed by addition of mobile phase, and the same is flushed through to make this completely wet and the precaution is taken to never run it dry. For the wet method the study of stationary phase with the eluent is prepared and then is poured into the column carefully [36, 37]. Examples of some phytochemicals isolated by our group in Jamia Hamdard, (Hamdard University), New Delhi, India, and other researchers using column chromatography are summarized in Table **2**.

Table 2. Examples of major phytochemicals isolated by column chromatography.

Phytoconstituents	Plant Name (part)	Mobile Phase	Stationary Phase	References
Lanostadienyl glucosylcetoleate		Chloroform		
Bengalensisteroic acid ester		Chloroform–methanol (97:3)		
Heneicosanyl oleate	*Ficus bengalensis* stem bark	Petroleum ether	Silica gel (60-120 mesh)	[37]
α-Amyrin acetate		Petroleum ether: chloroform (1:1)		
Lupeol		Petroleum ether: chloroform (1:1)		
Coriander lactone (2-α-n-heptatriacont-(Z)-3--n-1,5-olide)	*Coriandrum sativum* fruits	Petroleum ether	Silica gel (60-120 mesh)	[38]
Hydroxy coriander lactone (2α-n-tetracont-(Z,Z)-3, 26-dien-18α-ol-1,5-olide)		Chloroform		
Manglanostenoic acid A		Petroleum ether		
Manglanostenoic acid B	*Mangifera indica* bark	Petroleum ether-chloroform (9:1)	Silica gel (60-120 mesh)	[39]
Manglanostenoic acid C		Petroleum ether-chloroform (9:1)		
Manglanostenoic acid D		Chloroform-methanol(1:1)		
Cachemiridiol		Petroleum ether–chloroform (9:1)		
Continentalic acid	*Aralia cachemirica* root	Petroleum ether–chloroform (9:1)	Silica gel (60-120 mesh)	[40]
Tetrahydrocontinentic acid		Chloroform–methanol (49:1)		
Araliasesterterpenol		Chloroform–methanol (19:5)		
Mangolanostenoic acid A		Petroleum ether–chloroform (1:1)		
Mangosterolide	*Mangifera indica* stem bark	Petroleum ether–chloroform (1:1)	Silica gel (60-120 mesh)	[41]
Mangolanostendione		Petroleum ether–chloroform (1:3)		

Phytoconstituents	Plant Name (part)	Mobile Phase	Stationary Phase	References
bis-Isoflavonyldirhamnoside and artemisiaisoflavonyl glucosyldieste		Chloroform-methanol (99:1) and chloroform-methanol (95: 5)	Silica gel (60-120 mesh)	[42]
Stigmast-5,22-dien-3β-ol-21-oic acid-3β-glucopyranosyl-2'- octadec-9"-enoate; lanost-24-en-3β-ol-11-one-28-oic acid-21,23 α-olide-3β-D-glucopyranosyl-2'-dihydrocaffeoate-6'-decanoate; tricosan-14-on-1,4-olide-5-eicos-9'-enoate; and 3,11-dimethyldodecan-1,7-dioic acid-1-β-D-glucopyranosyl-6'-octadec-9"-enoate	Aerial parts of *Artemisia absinthium*	Petroleum ether-$CHCl_3$ (1:3); chloroform-methanol (97:3); chloroform-methanol (19:1); and chloroform-methanol (22:3), respectively	Silica gel (60-120 mesh)	[43]
Octatriacontenoic acid; norgadoleic acid; ketoberberine benzoate A; berberine phenoxide and ketoberberine benzoate B	*Berberis aristata* stem bark	Mixture of chloroform and methanol	Silica gel (60-120 mesh)	[44]
Swertiamarin	Aerial parts of *Enicostemma littorale*	*n*-Butanol-methanol (90:10)	Silica gel (60-120 mesh)	[45]
n-Hexadecanyl hexadecanoate; *n*-pentadecanyl octadec-9-enoate; *n*-hexadecanyl octadec-9-enoate; *n*-hexadecanyl-octadecanoate; and *n*-octadecanyl-octadecanoate	Seeds of *Cichorium intybus*	Mixture of chloroform and methanol	Silica gel (60-120 mesh)	[46]
n-decan-3-olyl pent-3'-en-1'-oate	Rhizomes of *Curculigo orchioides*	Chloroform–ethyl acetate (9:1)	Silica gel (60–120 mesh)	[47]
n-hexadec-9,11-dienyl cinnamate		Chloroform–ethyl acetate (4: 1)		
n-tridecanyl-hex-2',4'-dien-1'-oate		Chloroform-ethyl acetate (8: 2)		
n-heneitriacont-13-en-5,10-diol hex-2'-en-1'-oate		Chloroform–ethyl acetate (1: 1)		
1,5-diphenylpent-1-en-3-one	Aerial parts of *Escallonia illinita*	*n*-Hexane–ethyl acetate (8:2, v/v)	Silica gel (60–120 mesh)	[48]
4-(5-hydroxy-3,7-dimethoxy-4-*oxo*-4*H* chromen-2-yl)phenyl acetate		*n*-Hexane–ethyl acetate (8:2, v/v)		
Pinocembrin		*n*-Hexane–ethyl acetate (7:3, v/v)		
Kaempferol 3-*O*-methylether		*n*-Hexane–ethyl acetate (9:1, v/v)		
(3*S*,5*S*)-(*E*)-1,7-diphenylhept-1-ene-3,5-diol		*n*-Hexane–ethyl acetate (9:1, v/v)		
(3*S*,5*S*)-(*E*)-5-hydroxy-1,7-diphenylhept-1-en-3-yl acetate		*n*-hexane–ethyl acetate (4:6, v/v)		

(Table 2) cont.....

Phytoconstituents	Plant Name (part)	Mobile Phase	Stationary Phase	References
Nonacosanoic acid		*n*-Hexane-EtOAc (1:0 → 1:1).		[49]
Lupeol	*Vernonia glaberrima* leaves	*n*-Hexane-EtOAc (1:0 → 1:1)	(60–120 mesh)	
5-methylcoumarin-4-β-glucoside		CHCl$_3$-MeOH (1:0 → 0:1)		
4-Hydroxy-5-methylcoumarin		CHCl$_3$-MeOH (1:0 → 0:1)		
(3*S*,5*S*)-3,5-diacetoxy-1,7-*bis*(3,4,5-trimethoxyphenyl) heptane	Rhizomes of *Zingiber mekongense*	Me$_2$CO–hexane (1:1)	Silica gel (60–120 mesh)	[50]
Mahanimbine	Leaves of *Murraya koenigii*	Pet ether-chloroform (2:8)	Silica gel (60–120 mesh)	[51]
Lignan: 4'-*O*-demethylsuchilactone; phenolic compounds: rhododendrol; (-)-rhododendrin; sciadopytisin; ginkgetin; kayaflavone, (---secoisolariciresinol; suchilactone; three taxoids brevifoliol; 13-decinnamoyltaxchinin B; 10-deacetylbaccatin III	twigs (separated from the needles) of the Himalayan yew, *Taxus baccata*	Hexane, C$_6$H$_6$ and EtOAc	Silica gel (60–120 mesh)	[52]

2.3. Medium Pressure Liquid Chromatography (MPLC)

MPLC is a type of chromatographic separation procedure most appropriate for extensive research centre for the isolation of clean compounds from partially purified fractions. The procedure is accordingly complimentary to the flash chromatography; pressure range between 5-20 bars with appropriate flow rate, flash chromatography can be used to increase the speed without lowering the quality of the separation [53]. Flash chromatography (FC) is a type of MPLC; it provides fast, reliable and reproducible isolation and separation of bioactive phytochemicals. It is based upon column chromatography principles utilizing column packed with stationary phase such as silica gel (200 to 400 mesh) and mixtures of solvent as mobile phase. In flash chromatography, mostly 200 to 400 mesh size silica gel is used as stationary phase. For isolation of plant materials, fractionation of secondary metabolites is required for better and pure separation through flash chromatography. In this method of isolation and purification of phytochemicals, UV-visible spectroscopic detectors are utilized. The separation is guided by selection of appropriate absorption band from 200 to 800 nm. The collected fractions are evaluated and dried to constant weight [54, 55]. FC mainly utilized for isolation and separation of phytochemicals from higher medicinal plants [56 - 59]. It is also regularly used for purification of natural products also. Examples of some phytochemicals isolated by our group in Jamia Hamdard

(Hamdard University) New Delhi, India and other researchers using medium pressure liquid chromatography are summarized in Table **3**.

Table 3. Examples of major Phytochemicals isolated by medium pressure liquid chromatography.

Phytoconstituents	Plant Name (part)	Mobile Phase	References
Erythrocentaurin	Aerial parts of *Enicostemma littorale*	Ethyl acetate	[60]
23-*O*-β-*D*-glucopyranosyl-21-*O*-tigloyl-28-*O*-benzoyl-16,22-dimethoxygymnemagenin	*Gymnema sylvestre* leaf	Ethyl acetate	[61]
3-*O*-β-*D*-glucuronopyranosyl-16-*O*-acetyl-21-*O*-hydro-coumaroyl-16β,21β,23,29-tetrahydrox--oleanolic acid 28-*O*-β-*D*-glucopyranosyl ester		Ethyl acetate: methanol (98:2)	
3-β-*O*-*D*-glucopyranosyl-21-*O*-hydrocinnamoyl-16β,21β,23,29-tetrahydroxy-oleanolic acid 28-*O*-β-*D*-glucopyranosyl ester		Ethyl acetate: methanol (98:2)	
3-*O*-β-*D*-glucuronopyranosyl-21-*O*-hydrocinnamoyl-7β-hydroxygymnemagenin		Ethyl acetate: methanol (90:10)	
3-β-*O*-*D*-glucopyranosyl 3β,16β,23,28-tetrahydroxyolean-12-ene		Ethyl acetate: methanol (90:10)	
3α,21β,22α-trihydroxy-21,22-bis(2-methyl-1-oxobutoxy)-olean-15-en-23-methyl carboxylate-3yl-3-*O*-β-*D*-glucopyranosyl-(1→3)-*O*-β-*D*-glucuronopyranoside	*Gymnema sylvestre* leaf	Ethyl acetate	[62]
3α,7β,21β,22α-tetrahydroxy-21,22-bis (2-methyl-1-oxobutoxy)-olean-15-en-3yl-3-*O*-β-*D*-glucopyranosyl (1→3)-*O*-β-*D*-glucurono-pyranoside		Ethyl acetate: methanol (98:2)	
3α,7β,21β,22α-tetrahydroxy-21-(2-methyl-1-oxobutoxy)-22-[(2-methyl-1-oxobutenyl)oxy] olean-1--en-3yl-3-*O*-β-*D*-gluco-pyranosyl(1→3)O-β-D-glucurono-pyranoside		Ethyl acetate: methanol (98:2)	
3α,7β,21β,22α-tetrahydroxy olean-15-en-23,29-dioic acid-3-yl-3-*O*-β-*D*-glucopyranosyl (1→3)-*O*-β-*D*-glucurono-pyranoside		Ethyl acetate: methanol (90:10)	
3β,7β,21β,22α,23,28-hexahydroxy-21-(2-methyl-1-oxobutoxy)-22-[(2-methyl-1-oxob-tenyl)oxy]-olean-15-en-3-yl-3-*O*-β-*D*-glucopyranosyl (1→3)-*O*-β-*D*-glucurono-pyranoside		Ethyl acetate: methanol (90:10)	
Heteroclitin D	Stems of *Kadsurae interior*	Ethyl acetate (5-38%): pet ether	[63]
Polymethoxyflavones	Fruits of *Citrus reshni* and *Citrus sinensis*	Hexane and acetone (gradient program)	[64]

2.4. Preparative HPLC

Prep-HPLC is a sophisticated, relatively fast, accurate, versatile and robust technique for isolation phytochemicals from complex mixtures. Prep HPLC now days become a choice of method for isolation and purification of bioactive phytochemicals for structure elucidation and bioassay screening of new natural product in drug discovery [65]. In prep-HPLC column the particle size of stationary phase ranges from 3 to10 mm, the small particle size of stationary phase leads to higher column pressure (up to 3 to 4000 psi) which leads to efficient isolation. The main features of prep-HPLC are consistency and reproducibility in isolation of particular phytochemicals [66]. Reversed-phase HPLC is mostly used for isolation and purification of natural products. In this type of prep HPLC the stationary phase (for *e.g.* C_{18}, C_8 and polymeric polystyrene divinyl benzene) is more non-polar than the eluting solvents (for *e.g.* mixture of water and miscible organic solvents such as acetonitrile and methanol) [67]. Prior to performing prep-HPLC isolation of natural compounds, a systematic method development is required; the developed method should be validated, scale-up of parameters from analytical method to prep-HPLC were followed [68, 57]. In Table **4**, applications of prep-HPLC in isolation of natural compounds were summarized.

Table 4. Applications of prep-HPLC in isolation of natural products.

Plants	Phytochemicals	Instrument Conditions	References
Guierasere galensis	Galloylquinic acids	Column: RP-18e (250 × 10 mm i.d.); Mobile phase: Water: methanol: THF (90:10:0.25) and (80:20:0.25); Detection: 280 nm	[70]
Gleditsia japonica and *Gymnocladus chinensis*	Saponins	C18-µBondpak (300 × 24.4 mm i.d.); Methanol-water (varying percentages); Refractive index detector	[71]
Vicia faba	Procyanidins	Sephadex LH-20 column (580 × 25 mm i.d.); Sequential elution with ethanol, ethanol: methanol, methanol; Detection 280 nm	[72]
Taxus yunnanensis	Taxol	D1 (4000 × 200 mm i.d.) packed with 956 polymeric resin; Acetone: water (58:42); 228 nm	[73]
Vitex strickeri	Ecdysteroids	-	[74]
Bacitracin	Peptide components	Kromasil 5 C8 (250 × 16 mm I.D.); Mixture of methanol and acetonitrile	[75]

2.5. Preparative Gas Chromatography (Prep-GC)

Preparative gas chromatography (prep-GC) is a sophisticated isolation technique utilized for isolation and separation of essential oil components. This technique offers efficient and fast isolation of essential oil component. Till date there is no prep-GC equipment available commercially in market. For preparative separation of essential oil components, prep-GC must be modified as per requirement such as the injection port, column, split device and trap device of GC equipment [76]. Prep-GC becomes an important separation technique for separation of essential oil compounds; however, a heavier sample load and the large-diameter preparative column employed decreased the efficiency of prep-GC. The main disadvantages of prep-GC are lack of commercial prep-GC equipment, consumption of a large volume of carrier gas, the decomposition of thermolabile compound under high operation temperature, the difficulties of fraction collection and low production [77]. Prep-GC was utilized to separate five volatile compounds such as curzerene, β-elemene, curzerenone, curcumenol and curcumenone from methanolic extract of curcuma rhizome [78]. Prep-GC was also applied for the separation of natural isomers *e.g. cis*-asarone and *trans*-asarone were separated by using Prep-GC method from essential oil of *Acorus tatarinowii* [79].

2.6. Preparative TLC (Prep-TLC)

Preparative TLC (prep-TLC) is a chromatographic technique performed for isolation of natural compounds. This technique of isolation is simple and fast. The main difference between normal TLC to prep-TLC is the thick layer of stationary phase in it. For isolation of phytochemicals, first TLC method is developed and specific R_F is selected for isolation in preparative step. The developed chromatogram is scrapped with stationary phase and dissolved in solvents and filtered and dried under vacuum, and further used for other studies. This method is suitable for isolating milligrams to few grams of natural compounds. Prep-TLC is also a helpful technique for sample purification [80]. As compared with chromatography techniques, prep-TLC has the disadvantage of being difficult to automatize. By running small scale qualitative experiments, a large variety of eluents can be tested in a short time before the preparative work is done. When compared with preparative paper chromatography, thin layer chromatography is quicker and gives better separation. There have been many reported cases for separation of steroids, polyphenols and dyestuff successfully by using prep-TLC [81].

CONCLUDING REMARKS

Medicinal products derived from higher plants have been contributed to drug discovery and development over last century and continue to do so in present time too. The conventional isolation and separation techniques such as column chromatography and prep-TLC are time-consuming and require intensive lab work, and causes hindrance in drug development process. In recent years, due to advancement in isolation techniques such as prep-HPLC, MPLC, different types of counter-current chromatography, discovery of several preparative columns and prep-GC, the isolation and purification of bioactive natural products became easy and rapid. These advance and sophisticated isolation and purification systems also help in online identification and structural characterization when combined with advance detectors such as PDA and mass in case of UPLC, LC-MS and GC-MS, and thus these techniques make drug discovery and development from natural product rapid and cost effective.

ABBREVIATIONS

CC	Column chromatography
CCC	Counter-current chromatography
CPC	Centrifugal partition chromatography
DCCC	Droplet counter-current chromatography
DFCCC	Dual flow counter-current chromatography
HSCCC	High-speed or high performance counter-current chromatography
FC	Flash chromatography
MPLC	Medium pressure liquid chromatography
NCEs	New chemical entities
Prep-HPLC	Preparative high performance liquid chromatography
Prep-TLC	Preparative thin layer chromatography
Prep-GC	Preparative gas chromatography

CONSENT FOR PUBLICATION

Not applicable.

CONFLICT OF INTEREST

The author(s) confirms that there is no conflict of interest.

ACKNOWLEDGEMENTS

Declared none.

REFERENCES

[1]   Raina H, Soni G, Jauhari N, Sharma N, Bharadvaja N. Phytochemical importance of medicinal plants as potential sources of anticancer agents. Turk J Bot 2014; 38: 1027-35.
[http://dx.doi.org/10.3906/bot-1405-93]

[2]   Zahid Khan MA. Introduction and importance of medicinal plants and herbs. National Health Portal https://www.nhp.gov.in/introduction-and-importance-of-medicinal-plants-and-herbs_mtl

[3]   Fabricant DS, Farnsworth NR. The value of plants used in traditional medicine for drug discovery. Environ Health Perspect 2001; 109 (Suppl. 1): 69-75.
[PMID: 11250806]

[4]   Katiyar C, Gupta A, Kanjilal S, Katiyar S. Drug discovery from plant sources: An integrated approach. Ayu 2012; 33(1): 10-9.
[http://dx.doi.org/10.4103/0974-8520.100295] [PMID: 23049178]

[5]   Newman DJ, Cragg GM. Natural products as sources of new drugs from 1981 to 2014. J Nat Prod 2016; 79(3): 629-61.
[http://dx.doi.org/10.1021/acs.jnatprod.5b01055] [PMID: 26852623]

[6]   WHO. Quality control methods for medicinal plant materials. Geneva 1998.

[7]   Sasidharan S, Chen Y, Saravanan D, Sundram KM, Yoga Latha L. Extraction, isolation and characterization of bioactive compounds from plants' extracts. Afr J Tradit Complement Altern Med 2011; 8(1): 1-10.
[PMID: 22238476]

[8]   Mukherjee PK. Quality control of herbal drugs. 1st ed., Delhi: Business Horizons Pharmaceutical Publishers 2002.

[9]   Harborne JB. Phytochemical methods-A guide to modern technique of plant analysis. 3rd ed. London: Chapman and Hall 1998; pp. 109-45.

[10]   Trease GE, Evans WC. Pharmacognosy. 16th ed., London: Bailliere Tindall 2009.

[11]   Srivastava SK. Counter-current chromatography: Extraction technologies for medicinal and aromatic plants; Earth, environmental and marine sciences and technologies International Centre for Science and High Technology, ICS-UNIDO area Science Park Padriciano, 99, 34012 Trieste. Italy 2008; chapter 13: p. 209.

[12]   Altemimi A, Lakhssassi N, Baharlouei A, Watson DG, Lightfoot DA. Lightfoot phytochemicals extraction, isolation, and identification of bioactive compounds from plant extracts. Plants (Basel) 2017; 6(4): 1-23.
[http://dx.doi.org/10.3390/plants6040042] [PMID: 28937585]

[13]   Zhang Z, Pang X, Xuewu D, Jiang Y. Role of peroxidase in anthocyanin degradation in litchi fruit pericarp. Food Chem 2005; 90: 47-52.
[http://dx.doi.org/10.1016/j.foodchem.2004.03.023]

[14]   Popova IE, Hall C, Kubátová A. Determination of lignans in flaxseed using liquid chromatography with time-of-flight mass spectrometry. J Chromatogr A 2009; 1216(2): 217-29.
[http://dx.doi.org/10.1016/j.chroma.2008.11.063] [PMID: 19070866]

[15]   Skalicka-Woźniak K, Garrard I. Counter-current chromatography for the separation of terpenoids: a comprehensive review with respect to the solvent systems employed. Phytochem Rev 2014; 13(2): 547-72.
[http://dx.doi.org/10.1007/s11101-014-9348-2] [PMID: 24899873]

[16]   Berthod A, Maryutina B, Spivakov T, Shpigun B, Sutherland O, Ian A. Counter-current chromatography in analytical chemistry (IUPAC Technical Report). Pure Appl Chem 2009; 81(2): 355-87.
[http://dx.doi.org/10.1351/PAC-REP-08-06-05]

[17]   Ito Y, Bowman RL. Countercurrent chromatography: liquid-liquid partition chromatography without solid support. Science 1970; 167(3916): 281-3.
       [http://dx.doi.org/10.1126/science.167.3916.281] [PMID: 5409709]

[18]   Ito Y, Walter DC. High-speed counter current chromatography chemical analysis; J. New York: Wiley 1996.

[19]   Liu Y, Friesen JB, McAlpine JB, Pauli GF. Solvent system selection strategies in counter current separation. Planta Med 2015; 81(17): 1582-91.
       [http://dx.doi.org/10.1055/s-0035-1546246] [PMID: 26393937]

[20]   Ito Y, Goto T, Yamada S, *et al.* Application of dual counter-current chromatography for rapid sample preparation of N-methylcarbamate pesticides in vegetable oil and citrus fruit. J Chromatogr A 2006; 1108(1): 20-5.
       [http://dx.doi.org/10.1016/j.chroma.2005.12.070] [PMID: 16445929]

[21]   Tanimura T, Pisano JJ, Ito Y, Bowman RL. Droplet countercurrent chromatography. Science 1970; 169(3940): 54-6.
       [http://dx.doi.org/10.1126/science.169.3940.54] [PMID: 5447530]

[22]   Foucault AP. Centrifugal partition chromatography Chromatographic science series. CRC Press 1994; Vol. 68. ISBN 978-0-8247-9257-2.

[23]   Marchal L, Legrand J, Foucault A. Centrifugal partition chromatography: a survey of its history, and our recent advances in the field. Chem Rec 2003; 3(3): 133-43.
       [http://dx.doi.org/10.1002/tcr.10057] [PMID: 12900934]

[24]   Ito Y. Golden rules and pitfalls in selecting optimum conditions for high-speed counter-current chromatography. J Chromatogr A 2005; 1065(2): 145-68.
       [http://dx.doi.org/10.1016/j.chroma.2004.12.044] [PMID: 15782961]

[25]   Ogihara Y, Osamu I, Hideaki O, Kawai KI, Takenori T, Shoji S. Droplet counter-current chromatography for the separation of plant products. J Chromatogr A 1976; 128(1): 218-23.
       [http://dx.doi.org/10.1016/S0021-9673(00)84058-3]

[26]   Hostettmann K, Hostettmann KM, Otto S. Application of droplet counter-current chromatography to the isolation of natural products. J Chromatogr A 1979; 186: 529-34.
       [http://dx.doi.org/10.1016/S0021-9673(00)95273-7]

[27]   Hostettmann K, Hostettmann KM, Nakanishi K. Molluscicidal saponins from *Cornus florida* L. Helvetica 1978; 61(6): 1990-5.
       [http://dx.doi.org/10.1002/hlca.19780610607]

[28]   Kery A, Turiak G, Tetenyi P. Isolation of parthenolide by droplet counter-current chromatography. J Chromatogr A 1988; 446: 157-61.
       [http://dx.doi.org/10.1016/S0021-9673(00)94428-5]

[29]   Otsuka H, Ogihara Y, Shibata S. Isolation of coclaurine from *Zizyphus jujuba* by droplet counter-current chromatography. Phytochemistry 1974; 13: 9.
       [http://dx.doi.org/10.1016/0031-9422(74)85153-8]

[30]   Francis WG, Isaksen M. Droplet counter current chromatography of the carotenoids of parsley *Petroselinum crispum*. Chromatographia 1989; 27(11-12): 549-51.
       [http://dx.doi.org/10.1007/BF02258976]

[31]   Nasser LMN, Mazzolin PL, Hiruma LAC, Santos SL, Eberli NM, Brito MDA, *et al.* Preparative droplet counter-current chromatography for the separation of the new *nor-seco*-triterpene and pentacyclic triterpenoids from *Qualea parviflora*. Chromatographia 2006; 64(11-12): 695-9.
       [http://dx.doi.org/10.1365/s10337-006-0087-4]

[32]   Zhang S, Li L, Cui Y, *et al.* Preparative high-speed counter-current chromatography separation of grape seed proanthocyanidins according to degree of polymerization. Food Chem 2017; 219: 399-407.

[http://dx.doi.org/10.1016/j.foodchem.2016.09.170] [PMID: 27765243]

[33]   Zhang S, Cui Y, Li L, *et al.* Preparative HSCCC isolation of phloroglucinolysis products from grape seed polymeric proanthocyanidins as new powerful antioxidants. Food Chem 2015; 188: 422-9.
[http://dx.doi.org/10.1016/j.foodchem.2015.05.030] [PMID: 26041213]

[34]   Ali M. Text Book of Pharmacognosy. 2nd edn.., New Delhi: CBS Publishers & Distributors 2003.

[35]   Shusterman AJ, Patrick G. McDougal Glasfeld. Dry-column flash chromatography. J Chem Educ 1997; 74(10): 1222-3.
[http://dx.doi.org/10.1021/ed074p1222]

[36]   Zhang QW, Lin LG, Ye WC. Techniques for extraction and isolation of natural products: a comprehensive review. Chin Med 2018; 13(20): 20.
[http://dx.doi.org/10.1186/s13020-018-0177-x] [PMID: 29692864]

[37]   Naquvi KJ, Ali M, Ahamad J. Two new phytosterols from the stem bark of *Ficus bengalensis* L. J Saudi Chem Soc 2015; 19: 650-4.
[http://dx.doi.org/10.1016/j.jscs.2012.06.006]

[38]   Naquvi KJ, Ali M, Ahmad J. Two new aliphatic lactones from the fruits of *Coriandrum sativum* L. Org Med Chem Lett 2012; 2(1): 28.
[http://dx.doi.org/10.1186/2191-2858-2-28] [PMID: 22800677]

[39]   Ansari SH, Ali M, Naquvi KJ. New manglanostenoic acids from the stem bark of *Mangifera indica* var. "*Fazli.* J Saudi Chem Soc 2014; 18: 561-5.
[http://dx.doi.org/10.1016/j.jscs.2011.11.003]

[40]   Bhat ZA, Ansari SH, Ali M, Naquvi KJ. New phytoconstituents from the roots of *Aralia cachemirica* Decne. J Saudi Chem Soc 2015; 19: 287-91.
[http://dx.doi.org/10.1016/j.jscs.2012.03.004]

[41]   Ansari SH, Ali M, Naquvi KJ. New phytoconstituents from the stem bark of *Mangifera indica* var.*"Fazli.* India Drugs 2011; 48(11): 28-34.

[42]   Ahamad J, Naquvi KJ, Ali M, Mir SR. Isoflavone glycosides from aerial parts of *Artemisia absinthium* Linn. Chem Nat Compd 2014; 49(6): 696-700.
[http://dx.doi.org/10.1007/s10600-014-0807-1]

[43]   Ahamad J, Naquvi KJ, Ali M, Mir SR. New glycoside esters from the aerial parts of *Artemisia absinthium* Linn. Nat Prod J 2013; 3(4): 260-7.
[http://dx.doi.org/10.2174/2210315503041403281135181]

[44]   Ahamad J, Naquvi KJ, Ali M, Mir SR. New isoquinoline alkaloids from the stem bark of *Berberis aristata.* Indian J Chem B 2014; 53: 1237-41.

[45]   Ahamad J, Hasan N, Amin S, Mir SR. Swertiamarin contributes to glucose homeostasis *via* inhibition of carbohydrate metabolizing enzymes. J Nat Rem 2016; 16(4): 125-30.
[http://dx.doi.org/10.18311/jnr/2016/7634]

[46]   Najib S, Ahamad J, Mir SR. Isolation and characterization of fatty acid esters from the seeds of *Cichorium intybus.* Am J Phytomed Clin Therapy 2014; 2(4): 469-73.

[47]   Lakshmi N, Kumari S, Sharma Y, Sharma N. New Phytoconstituents from the Rhizomes of *Curculigo orchioides.* Pharm Biol 2004; 42(2): 131-4.
[http://dx.doi.org/10.1080/13880200490510964]

[48]   Montenegro I, Sánchez E, Werner E, *et al.* Isolation and identification of compounds from the resinous exudate of *Escallonia illinita* Presl. and their anti-oomycete activity. BMC Chem 2019; 13(1): 1.
[http://dx.doi.org/10.1186/s13065-019-0516-8] [PMID: 31355363]

[49]   Alhassan AM, Ahmed QU, Latip J, *et al.* Phytoconstituents from *Vernonia glaberrima* Wclw. Ex O. Hoffm. leaves and their cytotoxic activities on a panel of human cancer cell lines. S Afr J Bot 2018; 116: 16-24.

[http://dx.doi.org/10.1016/j.sajb.2018.02.391]

[50] Chareonkla A, Pohmakotr M, Reutrakul V, *et al.* A new diarylheptanoid from the rhizomes of *Zingiber mekongense.* Fitoterapia 2011; 82(4): 534-8.
[http://dx.doi.org/10.1016/j.fitote.2011.01.002] [PMID: 21238547]

[51] Dahiya J, Singh J, Kumar A, Sharma A. Isolation, characterization and quantification of an anxiolytic constituent - mahanimbine, from *Murraya koenigii* Linn. Spreng leaves. J Ethnopharmacol 2016; 193: 706-11.
[http://dx.doi.org/10.1016/j.jep.2016.10.014] [PMID: 27737817]

[52] Das B, Padma Rao S, Srinivas KVNS, Yadav JS. Lignans, biflavones and taxoids from Himalayan *Taxus baccata.* Phytochemistry 1995; 38(3): 715-7.
[http://dx.doi.org/10.1016/0031-9422(94)00678-M]

[53] Claeson P, Tuchinda P, Reutrakul V. Some empirical aspects on the practical use of flash chromatography for the isolation of biologically active compounds from plants. J Sci Soc Thailand 1993; 19: 73-86.
[http://dx.doi.org/10.2306/scienceasia1513-1874.1993.19.073]

[54] Still WC, Kahn M, Mitra A. Rapid chromatographic technique for preparative separations with moderate resolution. J Org Chem 1978; 43: 2923-5.
[http://dx.doi.org/10.1021/jo00408a041]

[55] Stevens WC Jr, Hill DC. General methods for flash chromatography using disposable columns. Mol Divers 2009; 13(2): 247-52.
[http://dx.doi.org/10.1007/s11030-008-9104-x] [PMID: 19140020]

[56] Dalsgaard PW, Potterat O, Dieterle F, *et al.* Noniosides E - H, new trisaccharide fatty acid esters from the fruit of *Morinda citrifolia* (Noni). Planta Med 2006; 72(14): 1322-7.
[http://dx.doi.org/10.1055/s-2006-951706] [PMID: 17051459]

[57] Mohn T, Plitzko I, Hamburger M. A comprehensive metabolite profiling of *Isatis tinctoria* leaf extracts. Phytochemistry 2009; 70(7): 924-34.
[http://dx.doi.org/10.1016/j.phytochem.2009.04.019] [PMID: 19467550]

[58] Berhow MA, Kong SB, Vermillion KE, Duval SM. Complete quantification of group A and group B soyasaponins in soybeans. J Agric Food Chem 2006; 54(6): 2035-44.
[http://dx.doi.org/10.1021/jf053072o] [PMID: 16536572]

[59] Weber P, Hamburger M, Schafroth N, Potterat O. Flash chromatography on cartridges for the separation of plant extracts: rules for the selection of chromatographic conditions and comparison with medium pressure liquid chromatography. Fitoterapia 2011; 82(2): 155-61.
[http://dx.doi.org/10.1016/j.fitote.2010.08.013] [PMID: 20804823]

[60] Hassan N, Ahamad J, Amin S, Mir SR. Rapid preparative isolation of erythrocentaurin from *Enicostemma littorale* by medium pressure liquid chromatography, its estimation by a validated HPTLC densitometric method and α-amylase inhibitory activity. J Sep Sci 2015; 38(4): 592-8.
[http://dx.doi.org/10.1002/jssc.201401030] [PMID: 25504557]

[61] Alkefai NH, Ahamad J, Amin S, Mir SR. Arylated gymnemic acids from *Gymnema sylvestre* R.Br. as potential α-glucosidase inhibitors. Phytochem Lett 2018; 25: 196-202.
[http://dx.doi.org/10.1016/j.phytol.2018.04.021]

[62] Alkefai NH, Sharma M, Ahamad J, Amin S, Mir SR. New olean-15-ene type gymnemic acids from *Gymnema sylvestre* (Retz.) R.Br. and their antihyperglycemic activity through α-glucosidase inhibition. Phytochem Lett 2019; 32: 83-9.
[http://dx.doi.org/10.1016/j.phytol.2019.05.005]

[63] Yu XX, Wang QW, Xu XJ, Lv W-J, Zhao M-Q, Liang Z-K. Preparative isolation of heteroclitin D from *Kadsurae Caulis* using normal-phase flash chromatography. J Pharm Anal 2013; 3(6): 456-9.
[http://dx.doi.org/10.1016/j.jpha.2013.07.004] [PMID: 29403855]

[64]   Uckoo RM, Jayaprakasha GK, Patil BS. Rapid separation method of polymethoxyflavones from citrus using flash chromatography. Separ Purif Tech 2011; 81: 151-8.
[http://dx.doi.org/10.1016/j.seppur.2011.07.018]

[65]   Hostettman K, Hostettman M, Marston A. Preparative chromatography techniques: applications in natural product isolation. Berlin, Germany: Springer-Verlag 1986; pp. 37-9.
[http://dx.doi.org/10.1007/978-3-662-02492-8]

[66]   Sarker SD, Latif Z, Gray AI. Natural Products Isolation. 2nd ed., Totowa, New Jersey: Humana Press 2005.
[http://dx.doi.org/10.1385/1592599559]

[67]   Euerby MR, Petersson P. Chromatographic classification and comparison of commercially available reversed-phase liquid chromatographic columns using principal component analysis. J Chromatogr A 2003; 994(1-2): 13-36.
[http://dx.doi.org/10.1016/S0021-9673(03)00393-5] [PMID: 12779216]

[68]   Mazzei JL, Avila LA. Chromatographic models as tools for scale-up of isolation of natural products by semi-preparative HPLC. J Liq Chromatogr Relat Technol 2003; 26: 177-93.
[http://dx.doi.org/10.1081/JLC-120017162]

[69]   Brandt A, Kueppers S. Practical aspects of preparative HPLC in pharmaceutical and development production. LC GC Eur 2002; 15(3): 147-51.

[70]   Bouchet N, Levesque J, Pousset JL. HPLC isolation, identification and quantification of tannins from *Guierasene galensis*. Phytochem Ann 2000; 11: 52-6.
[http://dx.doi.org/10.1002/(SICI)1099-1565(200001/02)11:1<52::AID-PCA482>3.0.CO;2-D]

[71]   Konoshima T, Yasuda I, Kashiwada Y, Cosentino LM, Lee KH. Anti-AIDS agents. 21: Triterpenoid saponins as anti-HIV principles from fruits of *Gleditsia japonica* and *Gymnocladus chinensis*, and a structure-activity correlation. J Nat Prod 1995; 58(9): 1372-7.
[http://dx.doi.org/10.1021/np50123a006] [PMID: 7494144]

[72]   Merghem R, Jay M, Brun N, Voirin B. Qualitative analysis and HPLC isolation and identification of procyanidins from *Vicia faba*. Phytochem Anal 2004; 15(2): 95-9.
[http://dx.doi.org/10.1002/pca.731] [PMID: 15116939]

[73]   Yang X, Liu K, Xie M. Purification of taxol by industrial preparative liquid chromatography. J Chromatogr A 1998; 813: 201-4.
[http://dx.doi.org/10.1016/S0021-9673(98)00332-X]

[74]   Zhang M, Stout MJ, Kubo I. Isolation of ecdysteroids from *Vitex strickeri* using RLCC and recycling HPLC. Phytochemistry 1992; 31: 247-50.
[http://dx.doi.org/10.1016/0031-9422(91)83046-N]

[75]   Pavli V, Kmetec V, Tanja T. Isolation of peptide components of bacitracin by preparative HPLC and solid phase extraction. J Liq Chromatogr Relat Technol 2004; 27: 2381-96.
[http://dx.doi.org/10.1081/JLC-200028153]

[76]   Wang H, Yang F, Xia Z. Progress in modification of preparative gas chromatography and its applications. Huaxue Tongbao 2011; 74(1): 3-9.

[77]   Ozek T, Demirci F. Isolation of natural products by preparative gas chromatography. Methods Mol Biol 2012; 864: 275-300.
[http://dx.doi.org/10.1007/978-1-61779-624-1_11] [PMID: 22367901]

[78]   Yang FQ, Wang HK, Chen H, Chen JD, Xia ZN. Fractionation of volatile constituents from *curcuma* rhizome by preparative gas chromatography. J Autom Methods Manag Chem 2011; 2011942467
[http://dx.doi.org/10.1155/2011/942467] [PMID: 21876660]

[79]   Zuo HL, Yang FQ, Zhang XM, Xia ZN. Separation of *cis*- and *trans*-asarone from *Acorus tatarinowii* by preparative gas chromatography. J Anal Methods Chem 2012; 2012402081

[http://dx.doi.org/10.1155/2012/402081] [PMID: 22448339]

[80] Nyiredy S. Chromatography: Thin layer (planar) preparative chromatography. Budakalasz, Hungary: Research Institute for Medicinal Plants 2000; p. 888.

[81] Ritter FJ, Meyer GM. Preparative thin-layer chromatography as an alternative for column chromatography. Nature 1962; 193: 941-2.
[http://dx.doi.org/10.1038/193941a0] [PMID: 14492518]

CHAPTER 5

Spectroscopic Techniques for the Structural Characterization of Bioactive Phytochemicals

Showkat R. Mir[1,*], **Tara Fuad Tahir**[2], **Javed Ahamad**[3], **Raad A Kaskoos**[4], **Naila Hassan Ali Alkefai**[5] and **Abdul Samad**[6]

[1] *Department of Pharmacognosy, School of Pharmaceutical Education and Research, Jamia Hamdard, New Delhi, India*

[2] *Faculty of Science and Health, Koya University, Kurdistan Region, Iraq*

[3] *Department of Pharmacognosy, Faculty of Pharmacy, Tishk International University, Kurdistan Region, Iraq*

[4] *Faculty of Pharmacy, Howler Medical University, Kurdistan Region, Iraq*

[5] *Collage of Pharmacy Department of Pharmacognosy & Phytochemistry University of Hafer Albatin Hafer Albatin, Kingdom of Saudi Arabia*

[6] *Department of Pharmaceutical Chemistry, Faculty of Pharmacy, Tishk International University, Kurdistan Region, Iraq*

Abstract: This chapter deals with the structural elucidation of natural products using UV-visible, FT-IR, NMR (1D and 2D) spectroscopy and Mass spectrometry. Key concepts associated with these techniques are introduced here. Various spectra of natural compounds have been included with a brief discussion of the functional groups and structural features that they reveal. The use of these spectroscopic techniques in drug discovery from natural products has been reviewed, highlighting the advantages of these techniques. The importance of each technique is discussed with suitable examples of natural products obtained from medicinal plants. Some of these techniques, such as FT-IR and NMR spectroscopy, are primarily used for identification purposes; while UV-visible spectroscopy and mass spectrometry are used for the purpose of analysis and structural elucidation. Recent advancements in the isolation techniques such as counter-current chromatography, supercritical fluid chromatography, preparative high-performance liquid chromatography (prep-HPLC), and preparative gas chromatography (prep-GC) have made the availability of novel natural compounds from plants possible for their structural elucidation and biological screening. Development of hyphenated techniques such as LC-NMR, UPLC-MS, and GC-MS have made simultaneous isolation and structural elucidation of natural products achievable. In this chapter, we have summarized basic principles of UV-visible, FT-IR, 1D and 2D NMR spectroscopy and mass spectrometry and their role in the determination of structures of natural compounds citing suitable examples.

* **Corresponding author Showkat R. Mir:** Department of Pharmacognosy, School of Pharmaceutical Education and Research, Jamia Hamdard, PO Hamdard Nagar, New Delhi, India 110 062; E-mail: showkatrmir@gmail.com

Javed Ahmad and Javed Ahamad (Ed.)

Keywords: FT-IR Spectroscopy, Mass Spectrometry, Natural Products, NMR Spectroscopy, UV-visible Spectroscopy, Structural Characterization.

1. INTRODUCTION

Phytochemistry deals with the study of various forms of secondary metabolites that are elaborated and accumulated in plants and also relate to their biosynthesis, turnover, metabolism, correlation and biological functions. Their isolation and characterization are important aspects of phytochemical studies [1]. Plant secondary metabolites are not only used as crude, raw and unmodified drugs, but they are also regarded to provide templates and starting materials for the production of various semi-synthetic drugs. For instance, diosgenin from *Dioscorea* species can be synthetically transformed to different steroids having anabolic, anti-inflammatory and oral contraceptive properties [2]. Phytochemicals that are used as therapeutic agents belong to classes such as alkaloids, glycosides, flavonoids, iridoids, terpenoids, resins, tannins, lignans, lipids, *etc* [3 - 7]. In recent decades, phytochemistry has played a central role in drug discovery and development processes. The enormous success of taxol has encouraged the scientific community worldwide to take up the research on drug discovery and development from plants. Recent technological advancements have opened various possibilities of phytochemical research to attain the new chemical entities as the drugs of future. The outlook of natural product chemistry has completely changed in the last few decades, which has witnessed explosive growth because of the advancement in extraction, isolation and characterization techniques. This has transformed the pace of drug discovery and development from natural substances. Development of separation techniques such as medium pressure liquid chromatography, preparative high-performance liquid chromatography (prep-HPLC), droplet counter-current chromatography (DCCC) and preparative gas chromatography (prep-GC), *etc.*, have greatly expedited and simplified the isolation and separation of complex mixtures of plant constituents that were thought to be inseparable earlier. Discovery of the powerful hyphenated techniques such as LC-NMR, LC-MS, and GCMS-MS has made the simultaneous isolation and structure elucidation of natural products possible [8, 9]. This chapter gives a preliminary overview of structural elucidation of natural products using UV-visible, FTIR, 1D and 2D NMR spectroscopy and Mass spectrometry.

2. STRUCTURAL ELUCIDATION OF PHYTOCONSTITUENTS

The step that precedes structural elucidation of natural compounds is their isolation and purification. Recent advancements in the isolation and purification techniques have made the process easy and fast. Soxhlet apparatus, Clevenger apparatus, supercritical fluid extractor, *etc.* are used for the separation of a specific mixture of phytochemicals from their matrices. It is followed by purification by chromatographic methods, liquid-liquid extraction, fractional distillation, solid-phase extraction, *etc.* These methods can be used repeatedly or in combination to attain required purity. Preliminary phytochemical screening consisting of physicochemical tests may also be employed to ascertain the nature of these compounds.

The preliminary characterization of phytochemicals is carried out, preferably by TLC analysis. If it yields a single spot on TLC plates in different mobile phases, it is considered fit for further characterization studies. Other parameters may also be used depending upon the nature of the isolates such as sharpness of melting/ boiling/ freezing point, refractive index, optical density, *etc.* Once the results of these preliminary studies show that the chemical compound is of desired purity and belongs to a specific class of phytoconstituents, the advanced techniques of structural determination are applied, such as UV, IR, NMR spectroscopy and mass spectrometry.

An already known compound can be identified by matching it's spectra with the reference spectra available in different libraries or databases. If the direct comparison can not be made, the spectra of related compounds reported earlier can be used for judicious structural comparison. On the other hand, for the characterization of a novel or an unknown compound, an extensive spectral analyses is performed [10 - 12].

2.1. UV-Visible Spectroscopy

Ultraviolet and visible spectroscopy is a technique to determine the absorption spectrum of a compound within a wavelength range of 200 to 800 nm. In this UV-visible region, a molecule absorbs the energy and undergoes through the changes in the electronic energy levels. Various chromophores within a molecule lead to the generation of a characteristic absorption spectrum. The absorption pattern of colourless solutions is measured in the range of 200 to 400 nm, while the coloured solutions are subjected to colourimetry in the range of 400 to 800 nm [13]. The spectra record wavelength of maximum and minimum absorption, as well as the intensity of absorption at a particular wavelength. For the identification purposes of many plant constituents, the UV-visible spectrum plays a very crucial role. The absorption spectra are critically valuable for the identification and determination of the chemical structure and analysis of natural compounds [14].

The electronic transitions in the molecules are classified as per the participating molecular orbitals. From the four possible transitions (n to π^*, π to π^*, n to σ, σ to σ*), only two can take place with light from the UV-visible spectrum for some biological molecules, *i.e.*, n to π* and π to π*. The n to σ and σ to σ* transitions do not lie energy-wise within the range of UV-visible spectrum and require higher energies. A chromophore is part of the molecular structure mainly responsible for the interaction with electromagnetic radiation. The chance of a photon to be absorbed by a matter is expressed by an extinction coefficient, which depends on the wavelength of the photon. If the light of certain intensity passes through a sample of appropriate transparency and the path length, the intensity keeps exponentially dropping along the pathway. According to the Beer Lambert's law, absorbance is proportional to the concentration of chromophores. The law does not hold well in the case of highly concentrated solutions [13, 14].

$$A = \varepsilon\, l\, c$$

Where A denotes absorbance, ε is the extinction coefficient, l is the path length and c denotes the concentration of a solution.

When the absorption spectra for a pure compound under defined conditions of solvent, concentration and temperature is obtained, it furnishes a set of values of ε (extinction coefficient) observed at a different wavelength in a solution of unit concentration (1 mole^{-1}) when the thickness of the layer travelled by the light is 1 cm of that particular solution. For a 1% weight by volume solution with the layer thickness of 1 cm, it is indicated as $\varepsilon\,{}^{1\%}_{1cm}$.

Table 1. Application of UV-visible spectroscopy in the analysis of natural products.

Spectroscopic method	Constituents	Wavelength
UV spectroscopy	Lobeline	249 nm
	Glycyrrhizinic acid	250 nm
	Allicin	254 nm
	Reserpine	268 nm
	Vinblastine	267 nm
	Tubocurarine chloride	280 nm
	Morphine	286 nm
	Vincristine	297 nm
	Vanillin	301 nm
	Colchicine	350 nm

(Table 1) cont.....

Spectroscopic method	Constituents	Wavelength
Visible spectroscopy	Ergot (total alkaloids)	530 nm by the use of *p*-dimethyl amino benzaldehyde reagent
	Morphine	442 nm by the nitroso reaction
	Reserpine	390 nm by treatment of alkaloid with sodium nitrite in dilute acid
	Tropic acid esters of hydroxytropanes	555 nm by Vitali-Morin reaction
	Anthraquinones	500 nm after treatment with alkali
	Capsaicin in capsicum	730 nm after reaction with phosphomolybdic acid and sodium hydroxide solution
	Cardiac glycosides Digitoxose moiety Lactone ring Ouabain	590 nm by Killer-Kiliani reaction 620 nm by reaction with m-dinitrobenzene 495 nm reaction with alkaline sodium picrate
	Cyanogenic glycosides	630 nm by the pyridine-parazolone colour reaction
	Procyanidins	545 nm
	Menthol in peppermint oil	500-579 nm by use of p-dimethyl amino benzaldehyde reagent
	Heperoside and isoquercitrin	425 nm with aluminium chloride and glacial acetic acid

British Pharmacopoeia utilizes UV-visible absorption characteristics as the standard for analysis of natural products such as lanatoside C, strychnine, brucine, benzylpenicillin, morphine, reserpine and tubocurarine chloride. Homoeopathic pharmacopoeia also utilizes UV-visible absorption characteristics as standards for quality control parameters of several medicinal herbs such as Aloe, Apocynum, Berberis, Ashoka, Syzygium, Terminalia and Viburnum. UV-visible absorption characteristics of most common natural products are summarised in Figs. (**1 - 4**) and Table **1**, which are highly helpful for the natural product chemists in the structural elucidation of phytochemicals.

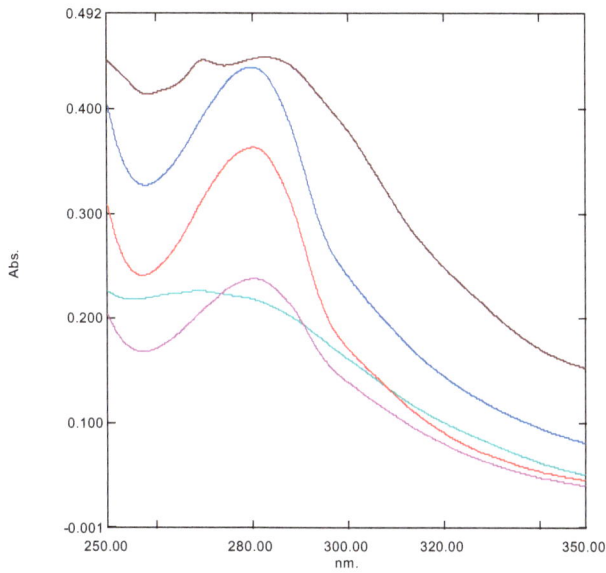

Fig. (1). UV absorption spectra of ethanolic extracts of different market samples of *Aloe vera;* Reference value 278, 310 nm [15].

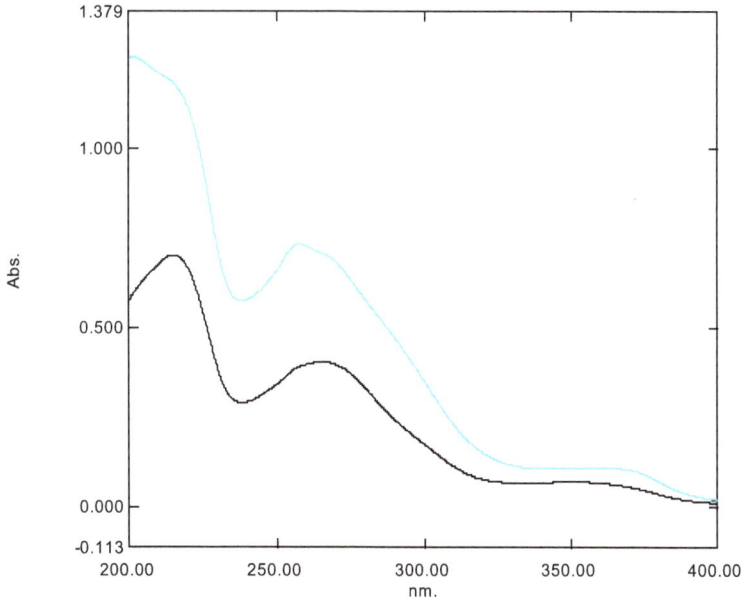

Fig. (2). UV absorption spectra of ethanolic extracts of different market samples of *Syzygium jambolanum*; Reference value 256 nm [15].

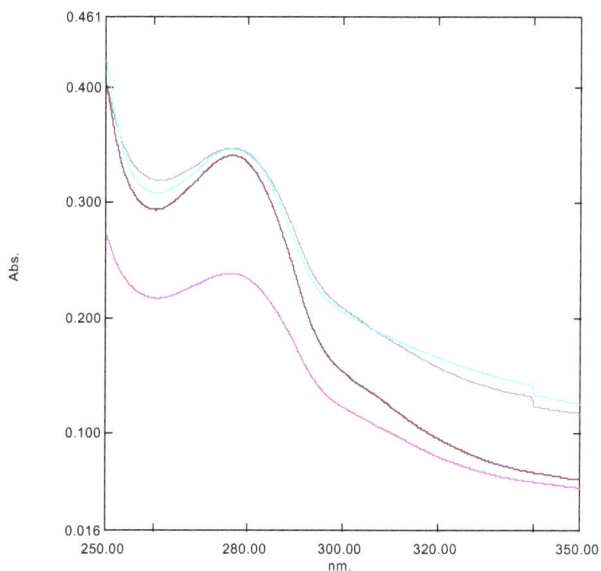

Fig. (3). UV absorption spectra of ethanolic extracts of different market samples of *Terminalia arjuna*; Reference value 270 nm [15].

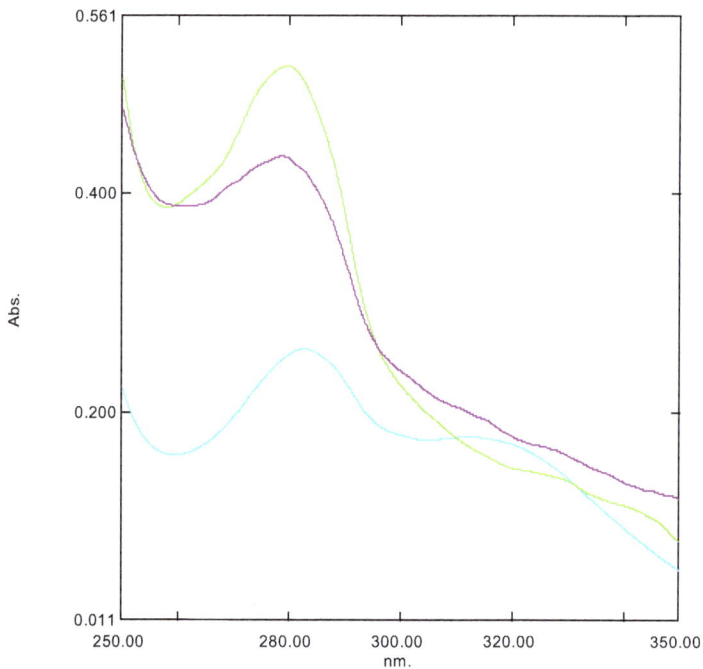

Fig. (4). UV absorption spectra of ethanolic extracts of different market samples *Viburnum prunifolium*; Reference value 272 nm [15].

2.2. Fourier Transform Infrared (FT-IR) Spectroscopy

FTIR is another important spectroscopic technique used to establish the presence of functional groups of the compounds. Functional groups can be identified by the characteristic vibrational frequencies in the IR spectrum. The IR spectrum is considered as one of the most reliable and simplest methods for knowing the structural framework of the novel compounds. IR spectroscopy deals with the infrared region of the spectrum ranging from 2.5 to 25 μm or 400 to 4000 cm^{-1}. The IR spectroscopy is often relied on for establishing the fingerprint of new and reported phytochemicals. The simplicity and reproducibility of IR spectrum, position this technique to be crucial for the complete identification of analytes [14 - 16].

IR spectroscopy is based on the fact that the molecules under study absorb the specific frequencies, which are characteristic of their molecular structure. For recording the IR spectrum of any compound, the dipole moment is a necessary requirement. In the range of 1450 to 600 cm^{-1} of the IR spectrum, it displays very complex peaks that are difficult to assign to the structural parts and due to this reason, this region is often called a fingerprint region. Likewise, the absorption band in the range of 4000 to 1450 cm arises because of the stretching vibrations of diatomic units and is called a group frequency region [16].

IR spectroscopy has been mainly divided into two main regions: (a) Diagnostic region from 3600 to 1200 cm that depicts clear information about the functional groups and contains fewer peaks; and (b) Fingerprint region from 1450 to 600 cm that depicts the peaks arising because of the vibrational excitations of most of the functional groups [16]. Table **2** summarises major peaks of different functional groups in natural products. Some examples of FTIR spectra are given below in Figs. (**5-8**).

Table 2. Characteristic IR frequencies of some classes of natural compounds.

Classes of natural compounds	Characteristic IR bands (in cm^{-1})
Alkanes	2940 (S), 2860 (M), 1455 (S), 1380 (M)
Alkenes	3050 (W-M), 1850 (W), 1650 (W-M), 1410 (W)
Alkynes	3300 (M), 2100-2270 (M)
Aromatic compounds	3050 (W-M), 2100-1700 (W), 1600, 1580, 1500 (W-M)
Acetylenes	3310 (M), 2225 (W), 2150 (W-M), 1300 (W)
Alcohols and phenols	3610 (W-M), 3600-2400 (br), 1420 (W-M)
Esters and lactones	1820-1680 (S)

(Table 2) cont.....

Classes of natural compounds	Characteristic IR bands (in cm^{-1})
Carboxylic acids	3520 (W), 3400-2500 (br, M), 1760 (S), 1710 (S)
Amines	3500 (M), 3400 (M), 3400-3100 (variable), 1610 (M)
Nitriles	2220-2260
Ketones, aldehydes (CO group)	1670-1740
Aldehydes (CH group)	2720-2820
Cyanides	2225 (W-S)
Isocyanates (NCO)	2232 (VS)

Where, S (strong), M (medium), W (weak), br (broad) and VS (very strong)

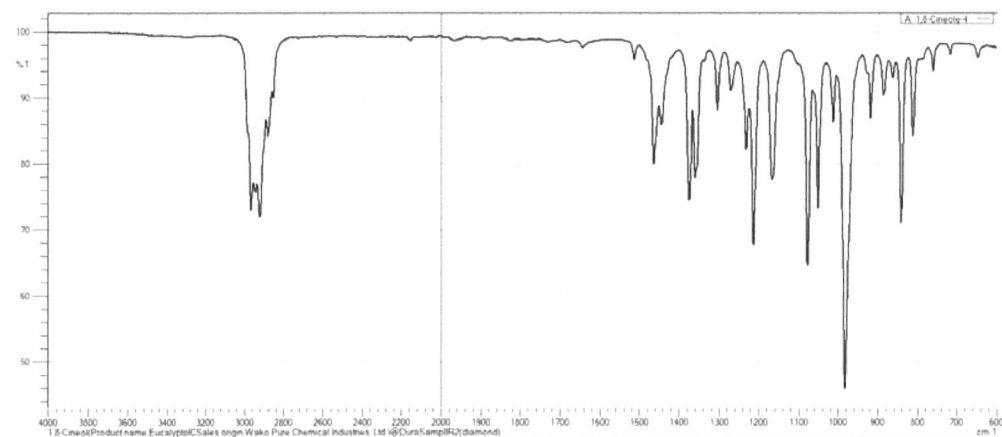

Fig. (5). Infra-Red spectrum of 1,8-Cineol.

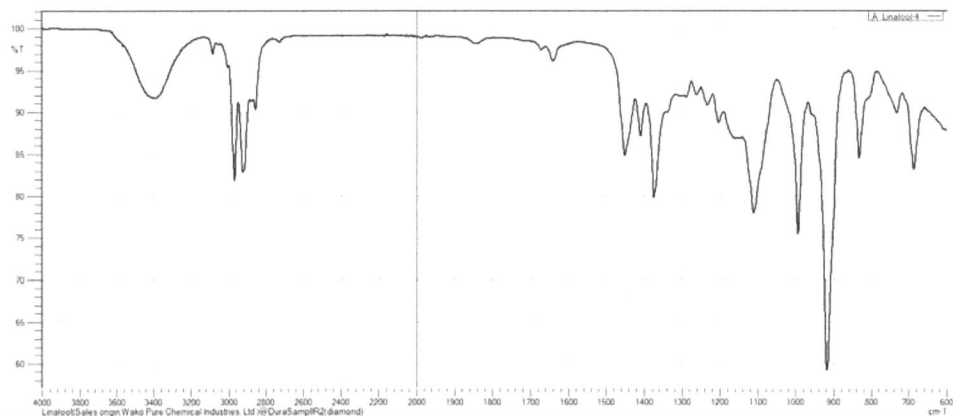

Fig. (6). Infra-Red spectrum of Linalool.

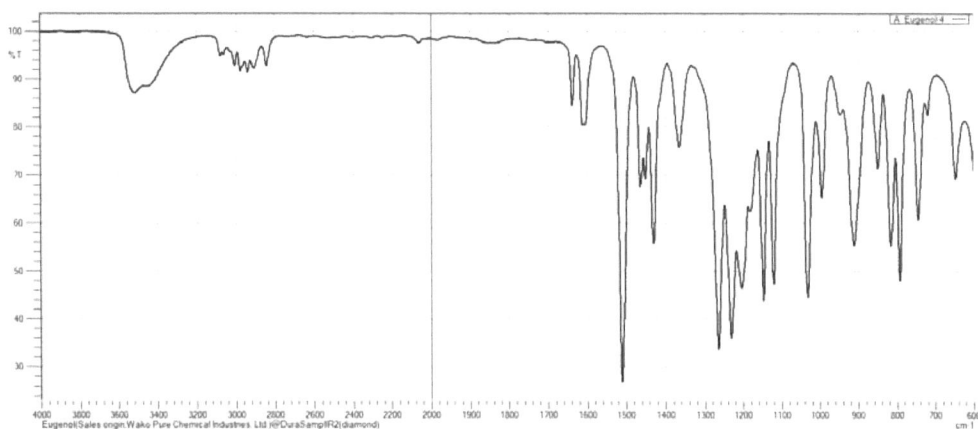

Fig. (7). Infra-Red spectrum of Eugenol.

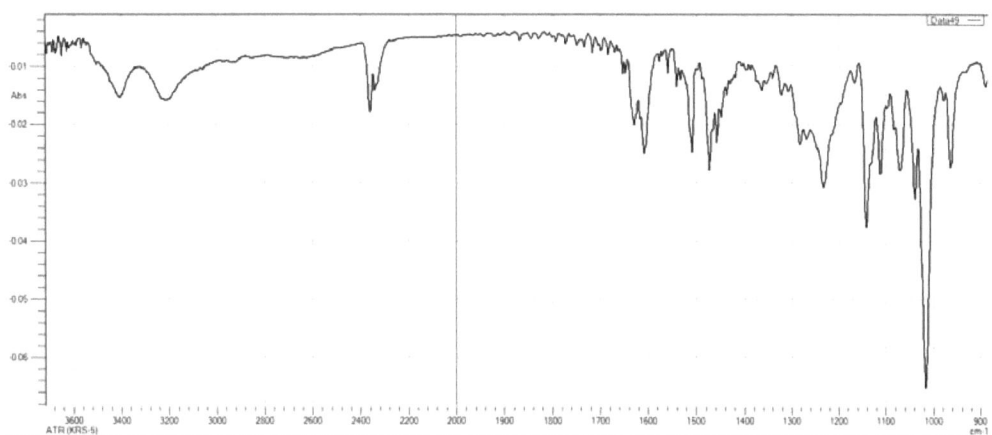

Fig. (8). Infra-Red spectrum of Catechin hydrate.

2.3. NMR Spectroscopy

NMR spectroscopy has evolved as an indispensable tool for the structural elucidation of compounds obtained from natural or synthetic origins. It is regarded as the most reliable technique for studying structures and transformations, as well as analysis and interactions of the chemical entities [16]. NMR is a non-destructive unbiased quantitative method, does not require separation or derivatization of samples. NMR results are highly reproducible. It helps in carrying out qualitative as well as quantitative estimation of compounds for semi-synthetic to natural molecules. Basically, two types of NMR are mostly used in the structural characterization of natural compounds. The first one is proton NMR (^{1}H NMR) and the second one is carbon NMR (^{13}C NMR). NMR spectroscopy is used as an important tool for the purpose of profiling of natural product extracts by providing accurate and precise composition and structural evidence for each of the component present [1, 17, 18].

Proton is present in virtually every molecule and the main isotope ^{1}H is contained in 98.95 percent abundance. Proton spectra are produced because its nucleus resonates with a frequency that is unique to its nature. The resonating frequency is extremely similar to the electronic environment, thereby imparting a particular NMR chemical shift to each 1H nucleus in a chemical compound. Chemical shifts and coupling constant provide extremely diagnostic information about the environment of resonating nuclei and the structure of chemical molecules. Thus, NMR spectroscopy has become a very effective tool for the structural elucidation of natural and synthetic compounds [19, 20].

The intensity of an NMR signal is largely influenced by excitation pulse, external magnetic field power, and temperature. The applied magnetic field and temperature determine the variations between the energy levels in Boltzmann's population. Thus, the excitation pulse determines the extent of the transition. Since the pulse used for ^{1}H nuclei excitations is the same, the transition range also remains the same for both. Interestingly, the NMR chemical change expressed by the resonant frequency differences of the unequal 1H nuclei is so small that it is expressed in part per million (PPM). The area under each peak in a ^{1}H NMR spectrum responds proportionally to the group of hydrogens present in the similar molecular environment of a compound [21]. Proton NMR spectroscopy determines the structure of an organic compound by measuring the magnetic moments of its hydrogen atoms.

The NMR spectrum depicts the differences in the chemical shift in PPM, which is the ratio of absolute frequency and frequency of the reference compound, Tetramethylsilane (TMS) [16, 22].

^{1}H NMR spectroscopy gives information regarding (a) the number of resonating protons which equals the number of non-equivalent protons, (b) the chemical shift of a proton, which indicates the chemical environment (offering shielding and deshielding), (c) integration value, indicates the number of equivalent H and (d) spin-spin coupling, which depends on the number of equivalent protons on the adjacent carbon. ^{1}H-^{1}H spin-spin coupling in proton NMR allows us to get the info about, (a) the chemically equivalent protons not showing spin-spin coupling to each other, (b) the resonance of a proton having n equivalent protons on the adjacent carbon splits into n+1 peaks with coupling constant J, (c) all the protons coupling to each other shall share the same coupling constant, (d) non-equivalent protons shall split a common proton independently [23].

Table 3. General regions of chemical shifts of different kinds of protons in ^{1}H NMR (0-10 ppm).

Chemical Classes	^{1}H NMR Chemical Shift (in δ Scale ppm)
Alkanes	0.85-0.95
Aliphatic acyclic protons	0-2.0
β-substituted aliphatic	1.0-2.0
Alkenes CH_3-C=C -CH=C	1.62-1.69 5.2-5.70
Acetylenes (HC≡C)	2.45-2.65
Aromatic protons Ar-H Ar-CH_3 Ar-CHO	6.60-8.0 2.25-2.50 9.70-10.0
Nitrogen compounds N-H N-CH_3 N-CHO	Variable 2.10-3.0 7.90-8.10
Alcohols (C-OH)	1.0-6.0 (variable)
Aldehyde (CHO)	9.0-12.0
Carboxylic acids (RCOOH)	10.0-12.0

^{13}C NMR spectroscopy highlights the nature of the carbon skeleton present in a chemical entity. ^{13}C NMR spectroscopy compliments ^{1}H NMR and the combination of the two techniques becomes a very powerful tool in the reign of structure characterisation of novel compounds from natural products such as terpenoids, glycosides, alkaloids or flavonoids. ^{13}C NMR detects the presence ^{13}C isotope, which is found in 1.1% abundance only. Because of the less abundance of ^{13}C nuclei larger amount of samples is required and longer time is also required for recording the ^{13}C NMR spectrum. The ^{13}C spectrum consists of larger chemical shifts ranging from 0 to 220 ppm [16]. The chemical shift values of some of the main carbon types are given in Table **4**.

Table 4. ^{13}C NMR peaks of major types of chemical classes.

Chemical Classes	^{13}C NMR Peaks from 0-220 ppm in δ Scale
Acyclic hydrocarbons CH$_3$ CH$_2$ CH	10-30 15-50 25-60
Alicyclic hydrocarbons	≈ 20
Alkenes	110-120
Alkynes	≈ 80
Aromatics	120-150
Alcohols (C-OH)	50-85
Ethers (C-O-C)	55-85
Acetals, Ketals (O-C-O)	90-110
Amines (C-NH$_2$)	20-70
Nitro (C-NO$_2$)	60-75
Aldehyde (CHO)	200-220
Ketone	190-220
Carboxylic acids (RCOOH)	160-185

^{1}H-^{13}C spin-spin coupling indicates the number of protons attached to ^{13}C nuclei (*i.e.*, Primary, secondary, tertiary carbon). ^{13}C spectra are measured with the ^{1}H-^{13}C coupling "turned off" (broadband decoupled).

In this mode, all ^{13}C resonances appear as singlets. DEPT spectra (Distortionless Enhancement by Polarization Transfer) is a type of ^{13}C NMR spectroscopic technique that allows the determination of the number attached to a carbon. Only CH determination can be made by using DEPT90. DEPT-135 defines the positive resonance of CH and CH$_3$, while the negative resonances define CH$_2$ [24]. Table **5** outlines the scope and the use of 2D NMR spectroscopy in the structural elucidation of natural or synthetic drugs.

Table 5. Major types of 2D NMR spectroscopy and their scope in the elucidation of chemical structure.

2D NMR Types	Scope of Method
HSQC (Heteronuclear Single Quantum Coherence)	The HSQC spectrum demonstrates resonances originating from couplings of $_1$J$_{CH}$ between the 13C nuclei and protons connected to their respective atoms. It allows the identification of chemical categories of all CH, CH$_2$ and CH$_3$ groups.
COSY (Correlation spectroscopy)	The COSY spectrum usually shows homonuclear correlations (spin couplings) between three bonds (^{3}J$_{HH}$) separated by vicinal carbons. It allows for the recognition of adjacent carbon atoms linked by a chemical bond.

(Table 5) cont.....

2D NMR Types	Scope of Method
HMBC (Heteronuclear Multiple-Bond Coherence)	The HMBC spectrum reveals heteronuclear correlations between ^{1}H and 13C (^{15}N) nuclei separated by two or three chemical bonds which allow users to detect *"fuzzy"* fragments around a given C or N atom.
TOCSY (Total Correlation Spectroscopy)	In general, TOCSY helps one to get sub-spectra for various sequences of coupled protons in a molecule.
NOESY (Nuclear Overhauser Enhancement Spectroscopy)	The NOESY shows the coupling between spatially separated hydrogen atoms by a distance of more than 5 angstroms, which is used to decide the stereochemistry of an elucidated structure, as well as to explain the positions of certain substituents if HMBC and COSY data do not allow this to be done.

2.4. Mass Spectrometry

Due to its high accuracy in assessing molecular mass, mass spectrometry is an important method for the structural assessment of natural products. Mass spectroscopy just requires samples in micrograms to be evaluated and gives reliable and reproducible results. Mass spectroscopy is being used to obtain patterns of fragmentation and molecular mass for samples of either synthetic or natural origin [16, 25, 26]. Mass spectrometry is also commonly used to evaluate substances with the previously reported mass spectrum, and to analyze new unknown compounds as well. The catalogue of the identified compounds is measured and compared for an already known compound with the spectrum of the compound in question. In order to classify and determine the molecular structure of the newly discovered molecule, UV, IR, NMR and Mass spectrometry techniques are used in combination to arrive at a plausible structure [26].

Samples are ionized in mass spectroscopy by allowing them to travel through an analyser where they are detected based on the mass to charge ratio. The vapor of the sample is made to disperse in the low-pressure system of the mass spectrometer, which ionizes the compound with sufficient energy and allows it to be fragmented. This allows positive ions to be produced that are stimulated by the applied magnetic field and are moving according to the mass to charge ratio. The continuous separation and quantification process can be accomplished by coupling the liquid chromatography (LC) techniques with mass spectrometry (MS). That is why LC is now paired with MS to identify and characterize natural compounds expeditiously and efficiently [27 - 29]. Owing to recent technological developments, the introduction of multidimensional LC systems based on the sequential separation in the biphasic column consisting of stationary phases with different characteristics has improved the efficiency of LC-MS systems considerably. The recently introduced multidimensional protein identification technology (MudPIT) in the area of proteomics [29, 30] is the amalgamation of two-dimensional LC and multidimensional protein recognition techniques. The multidimensional RP ion-exchange LC-MS-MS method was used by Washburn *et al.* and Walters at al. for qualitative protein analysis in a complex mixture [31, 32]. Walter *et al.*, have designed a two-dimensional RP-RP NANO-UPLC device in Manchester, United Kingdom. Well into the sense of RP chromatography in both dimensions and with specific pH values, this method has been designed for high reproducibility and an excellent separation performance [33 - 36].

MALDI-TOF Mass Spectrometry: MALDI-TOF MS (matrix-assisted laser desorption/ ionization-time of flight mass spectrometry) has proven to be very effective for the detection and characterization of secondary metabolites [37]. It became one of the first choice methods in protein and amino acid identification and characterization because of its advantages such as highly sensitive, speed of analysis, robustness and the prevalence of single charged ions [38 - 40].

ESI MS Mass Spectrometry

Electron spray ionization MS is now being used as a proven method for evaluating proteins and peptides in food and natural products and for their structural characterization.

LC system is used for the separation and ESI MS/MS is used for identification and quantification of proteins and high molecular weight natural products. The tandem mass spectrometer is commonly used as a triple quadrupole MS/MS, which consists of a vacuum chamber containing two quadrupole mass filters separated by a collision cell between both the quadrupoles [39]. Natural substances in LC-ESI-MS get protonated with the ESI source and form multiply charged ions with mass to charge ratios ranging from 200 to 2000 amu and then during collision-induced dissociation, different degrees of protonation could coexist and several peaks could be observed for each peptide because peptide bonds are relatively weak.

The detection of particular transitions with the most powerful stimulus for the fragments is, therefore, crucial for the recognition of proteins. The fragments are isolated in ESI MS/MS using the m/z ratio [35, 41]. This selected reaction monitoring (SRM) method, also referred to as Multiple Reaction Monitoring (MRM), has been proved reproducible and effective in protein and amino acids' quantification across numerous laboratories.

Recently, with the assistance of the use of a hybrid three-fold quadrupole and a linear ion trap devise, the MRM method emerged as a crucial tool for improving the sensitivity, precision, and scanning speed of mass spectrometers since it enables secondary fragmentation within the 3rd quadrupoles by trapping ions in daughters for a positive time frame before they are detected [35]. Fortin *et al.* have shown that MRM, combined with liquid chromatography, contributed to three to fivefold improvements in serum prostate-specific level detection and quantification limits [42].

3. CASE STUDIES: SOME EXAMPLES OF STRUCTURAL CHARACTERIZATION OF NATURAL PRODUCTS

3.1. Erythrocentaurine (EC)

Medium pressure chromatography using a silica gel was performed for the ethyl acetate fraction of the methanolic extract of *Enicostemma littorale* (Gentianaceae). After spraying with anisaldehyde-sulphuric acid reagent, a bright pink spot appeared on TLC plates for hexane ethyl-acetate (90:10 v/v) eluents. This compound was then isolated as a colorless needle (which turn brown on exposure to light). It was characterized on the basis of data given below and in Table **6**.

Table 6. NMR spectroscopic data of erythrocentaurin in methanol.

Position	^{1}H NMR(500 MHz)	^{13}C NMR(125MHz)	DEPT
1	-	165.4	C
3	4.51 dd (5.6,6.0)	66.77	CH$_2$
4	3.53 dd (5.6,6.0)	24.58	CH$_2$
5	-	126.86	C
6	-	132.59	C
7	8.01 d (7.6)	135.62	CH
8	7.58 dd (7.6,7.6)	127.88	CH
9	8.31 d (7.6)	138.43	CH
10	-	141.17	C
11	10.17 s	191.95	CH

Chemical shift values (δ) expressed in ppm, coupling constants in Hertz are provided in parentheses.

R_f value: 0.63 (hexane-ethyl acetate, 1:3)

m.p.: 137-139 °C (lit. 140-141 °C)

UV λ_{max} (MeOH): 224, 291 nm

IR n_{max} (KBr): 3364, 2920, 1724, 1695,1585, 1463,1400,1290, 1116 cm^{-1}

^{1}H and ^{13}C NMR: (Table **6**)

-ve ESI-MS *m/z*: 175 [M-H]$^{-}$ $C_{10}H_7O_3$.

The compound's UV spectrum, showing maxima in MeOH at 224 and 291 nm, indicated an aromatic chromophore. The IR spectrum showed vibrations of carbonyl at 1724 and 1695 cm^{-1}, respectively, for unsaturated δ-lactone and conjugated aldehyde. The characteristic absorption peak appeared at 1585 cm^{-1} for the aromatic moiety. The ESI-MS measured, mass spectrum showed an[M-H] ion at m/z 175, which was in line with the molecular formula $C_{10}H_8O_3$. The ^{1}H NMR spectrum of isolated compound displayed three ortho-meta coupled downfield signals at δ$_H$ 8.01 (1H, d, *J* = 7.6 Hz), 7.58 (1H, dd, *J* = 7.6, 7.6 Hz) and 8.31 (1H, d, *J* = 7.6 Hz) assigned to H-7, H-8, and H-9 aromatic protons, respectively. It also exhibited two-proton double-doublets at δ$_H$ 4.51 and 3.53 (*J* = 5.6, 6.0Hz, each), ascribed to H$_2$-3 and H$_2$-4 methylene protons. A singlet at δ$_H$ 10.17 was typical of an aldehydic proton. ^{13}CNMR and DEPT experiments exhibited 10 carbons consisting of two methylenes (including one oxygenated ethylene), four methine (including one aldehyde) and four quaternary carbons. On the basis of the above discussion, the structure of the compound was elucidated as erythrocentaurin (Fig. **9**) [11].

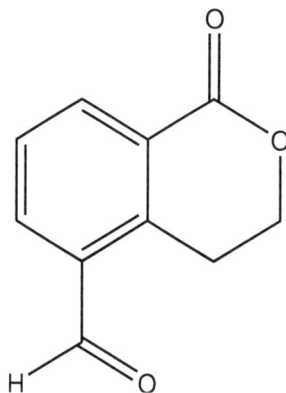

Fig. (9). Chemical structure of Erythrocentaurin (EC).

3.2. Octatriacontanoic Acid (OA)

The **octatriacontanoic acid** (OA), was isolated by column chromatography of the methanolic extract of stem bark of *Berberis aristata* using chloroform: methanol (93:7) as eluent. It was purified as a colourless amorphous powder from methanol-acetone (1:1), **(0.461 mg,0.05% yield).**

R_F value: 0.60 (chloroform- methanol, 97:3)

m.p.: 52-53° C

UV λ_{max} (MeOH): 207 nm (log ε 3.1)

IR ν_{max} (KBr): 3373, 2923, 2853, 1710, 1640, 1463, 1271, 1170, 722 cm^{-1}

^{1}H NMR (CDCl$_3$): δ 5.68 (1H, m, H-22), 5.34 (1H, m, H-21), 2.31 (2H, m, H$_2$-2), 2.05 (4H, brs, H$_2$-20, H$_2$-23), 1.61 (4H, m, 2×CH$_2$), 1.28 (58 H, brs, 29×CH$_2$), 0.89 (3H, t, J= 6.1 Hz, Me-38)

^{13}C NMR (CDCl$_3$): δ 177.62 (C-1), 129.77 (C-21), 127.78 (C-22), 56.06 (C-2), 31.17 (C-20), 31.69 (C-23), 31.30 (CH$_2$), 29.43 (21×CH$_2$), 29.08 (2×CH$_2$), 24.61 (CH$_2$), 23.05 (CH$_2$), 22.40 (CH$_2$), 13.77 (Me-38)

+ve FAB MS m/z (rel. Int.): 562 [M]$^+$ (C$_{38}$H$_{74}$O$_2$) (15.4), 547 (9.1), 337 (22.1), 311 (26.3), 251 (28.6), 225 (29.2)

The compound (**OA**) gave effervescence with NaHCO$_3$ solution and decolourized bromine water. The typical absorption bands of its IR spectrum were due to its aliphatic nature (722 cm^{-1}) and the carboxylic group (3373, 1710 cm^{-1}). It has been found to have a molecular weight m/z 562 on the basis ^{13}C NMR and mass spectra in accordance with the molecular formula C$_{38}$H$_{74}$O$_2$ of an aliphatic acid. The formula indicated two double bonds; one in an olefinic bond and the other in a carboxylic bond. Olefinic binding of C21 was shown in the diagnostic ion peaks at m/z 225, 337[C$_{22}$–C$_{23}$fission]$^+$ and 251, 311[C$_{20}$-C$_{21}$ Fission]$^+$. The ion peak of m/z 547[M-Me]+ followed the long aliphatic character of the OA chain. The ^{1}HNMR spectrum of OA displayed two vinyl H-22 and H-21 protons at δ 5,68 and 5,34 downfield multiplets, each assimilated for one proton. The methylene H2-2-2 protons adjacent to the vinyl linkage are assigned a two-proton multiplet at μ 2.31. H$_2$-20 and H$_2$-23 methylene protons next to the vinyl contact have been due to a 4-proton wide singlet at δ 2.05. The remaining protons of methylene resonated as four-proton and fifty-eight proton wide signals raised on δ 1.61 and 1.28, respectively. The residual carbons of methylene ranged from δ 56.06 to 22.40, while the dominant methyl carbon Me-38 was estimated to be at δ 13.76. The compound structure of octatriacont-21-en-1-oic acid was elucidated based on the above discourse, (Fig. **10**) [18].

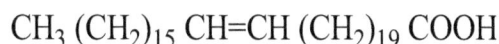

$$CH_3 \ (CH_2)_{15} \ CH=CH \ (CH_2)_{19} \ COOH$$

Fig. (10). Chemical structure of Octatriacontenoic acid (**OA**).

3.3. Norgadosic Acid (NA)

Norgadosic acid has been isolated using chloroform-methanol (91:9) as eluent in the column chromatography of methanolic extract of *Berberis aristata* stem bark. It yielded colourless crystals after recrystallization by methanol: acetone (1:1), and yielded(0.825 mg., 0.08%).

R_f value: 0.69 (chloroform-methanol, 91:09)

m.p.: 40-41° C

UV λ_{max} (MeOH): 206, 263nm (log ε 2.1, 1.1)

IR n_{max} (KBr): 3380, 2923, 2852, 1710, 1640, 1463, 1335, 1270, 1090, 720 cm^{-1}

^{1}H NMR (CDCl$_3$): δ 5.50 (1H, m, H-7), 5.35 (1H, m, H-8), 2.77 (2H, m, H$_2$-2), 2.29 (2H, m, H$_2$-6), 2.04 (2H, m, H$_2$-9), 1.62 (2H, m, H$_2$-3), 1.27 (20H, brs, 10×CH$_2$), 0.88 (3H, t, J =6.1 Hz, Me- 18)

^{13}C NMR (CDCl$_3$): δ 177.47 (C-1), 129.95 (C-7), 127.91 (C-8), 56.05 (C-2), 33.78 (CH$_2$), 31.67 (CH$_2$), 31.64 (CH$_2$), 29.42 (4×CH$_2$), 29.07 (CH$_2$), 28.90 (CH$_2$), 26.99 (CH$_2$), 26.99 (CH$_2$), 25.46 (CH$_2$), 24.61 (CH$_2$), 22.39 (CH$_2$), 13.77 (Me-18)

+ve FAB MS *m/z* (rel. Int.): 282 [M]$^+$ (C$_{18}$H$_{34}$O$_2$) (33.6), 167 (42.3), 141 (47.0), 115 (78.5)

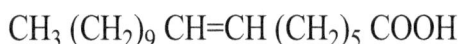

$$CH_3 \, (CH_2)_9 \, CH{=}CH \, (CH_2)_5 \, COOH$$

Fig. (11). Chemical structure of Norgadosic acid.

The IR spectrum of the carboxylic groups (1710 cm^{-1}), unsaturation (1640 cm 1) and aliphatic chain (720 cm^{-1}) displayed characteristic absorption belts. When treated with NaHCO$_3$ solution, it yielded effervescence and decolorised the bromine water. Its IR spectrum exhibited characteristic absorption bands for the carboxylic group (1710 cm^{-1}), unsaturation (1640 cm^{-1}) and aliphatic chain (720 cm^{-1}). Their molecular weight has been identified as m/z 282 by ^{13}C NMR and the mass spectrum corresponding to the aliphatic acid having molecular formula C$_{18}$II$_{34}$O$_2$. Two double bond equivalents were indicated that each was adjusted for carboxylic and vinyl. Diagnostical value of ionic peaks appearing at 140, 141 and 167 suggested C8–C9 and C6–C7 fission, which was due to the vinyl linkage at

C7. At δ 5.50 and 5.35 the ¹H NMR, NA spectrum displayed two different downfield signals each granting vinyl protons H-7 and H-8. Three two multiple protons at δ 2.77, 2.29 and 2.04 tended to be somewhat downfield in comparison to the usual methylene proton signals and were due to protons of H-2 andH-7 and H-9 adjacent to olefinic association. Around δ1.62 (2 H) and 1.27 (20 H), the rest of the protons emerged. Me-18 primary methyl protons were interpreted in a three-proton triplet at δ 0.88 (J = 6.1 Hz).

At δ 177.47 (C-1) and δ 129.95 (C-7) and 127.91 (C-8), the ¹³C NMR of NA spectrum showed significant signals of carboxyl carbon. The carbon of methylene resonated between δ 55.0 –22.39, and the carbon of methyl Me-18 was at δ 13.77. It has been suggested to be a C18 acid isoform by different physical NA from that of oleic acid and vaccenic acid. The compound composition was described as octadec-7-enoic acid (Fig. **11**) based on the above definition [18].

3.4. Isoalantolactone (IL)

The normal phase column chromatography of methanol extract from *Inularacemosa* roots, yielded compound **IL** as a white amorphous powder with hexane-ethyl acetate (70:30 v/v) eluents. Fig. (**12**) shows its structure. Physical condition: amorphous white powder, RF 0.81 (toluene-chloroform-ethanol, 8:8:2); yield 0.22%.

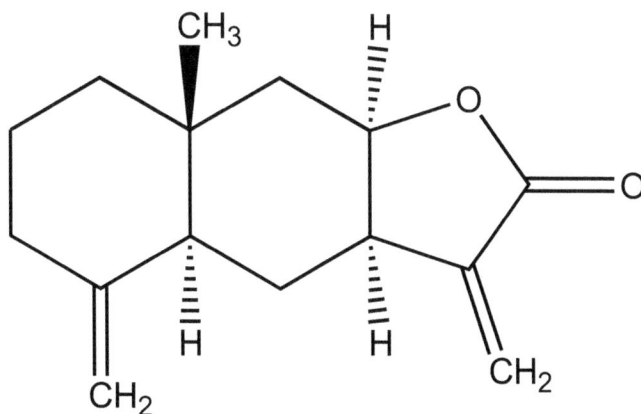

Fig. (12). Chemical structure of compound Isoalantolactone.

UV λ_{max} (MeOH): 214, 265 nm

FTIR (KBr) v_{maxx}: 2924, 1737, 1643, 1444, 1261, 948 cm⁻¹

^{1}H and ^{13}CNMR (CDCl$_3$): See Table 7

Table 7. NMR data of Isoalantolactone.

Position	^{1}H MNR	^{13}C NMR	DEPT-135
1	1.25 m	40.5	CH$_2$
2	1.54 m	22.6	CH$_2$
3	2.32 m	41.7	CH$_2$
4	-	149.4	C
5	2.14 dd (1.0, 4.5)	46.5	CH
6	1.81 m	27.4	CH$_2$
7	2.95 m	39.5	CH
8	4.47 dd (1.0, 4.0)	76.4	CH
9	1.70 m	42.6	CH$_2$
10	-	34.8	C
11	-	142.2	C
12	-	170.6	C
13	6.09 br s, 5.56 br s	120.0	CH$_2$
14	0.75 s	17.6	CH$_3$
15	4.74 d (1.0), 4.41 d (1.0)	106.5	CH$_2$

+ve ES-MS m/z (rel. int.): 233 [M + 1]$^+$C$_{15}$H$_{21}$O$_2$ (69), 215 (92), 187 [M - CO$_2$]$^+$ (100)

The absorption bands of the carbonyl group and the olefinic links in the FTIR spectrum were found at 1737 cm^{-1} and (1643, 1444 cm^{-1}), respectively. The molecular weight of IL was established to be 232, compatible with the molecular formula C$_{15}$H$_{20}$O$_2$, based on ^{13}C/DEPT and mass spectra. The formula represented the presence of six double bond equivalents, three of which were configured in a tricyclic system, two in vinyl contacts and the rest in a carbonyl group. Its +ve ES-MS exhibited a quasi-molecular ion peak at m/z233 [M + 1]$^+$, a fragment ion peak at m/z 215 [C$_{14}$H$_{15}$O$_2$] $^+$ and a base peak at m/z 187 [M-CO$_2$]$^+$.The ^{1}H NMR spectrum of **IL** showed typical signals for the protons associated with two exocyclic vinylic linkage at δ 6.09 and 5.56 (both br s, 1H) and 4.74 and 4.41 (both d, J = 1.0 Hz, 1H) ascribed correspondingly to H$_2$-13a, H$_2$-13b, H$_2$-15a and H-15b protons. Signals resonated at 149.4(C-4), 106.5(C-15), 142.2(C-11) and 120.0 (C-13) for vinyl carbons. The carbonyl carbon signals at δ 170.6 (C-12) supported the presence of the alpha lactone ring that had not been saturated. The presence of eudesmolide mode was supported by a double double-doublet signal at δ 4.47 (J= 1.0, 4.0 Hz, H-8) at ^{1}H NMR and a resonated at δ 76.4 (CH-8). The tertiary methyl group (H 3-14) has been assigned a 3 Proton singlet at δ 0.75. The presence of 15 Carbon resonances consisting of 4 quaternary carbons, 3 methine carbons, 7 Methylene carbons and 1 Methyl carbon has been shown through a carefully studied ^{13}C/DEPT NMR Data. Comparison of ^{1}H/^{13}C NMR and mass and the melting point of IL with that of isoalantolactone was found to be in good alignment with the second major Eudesmalactone recorded for different Inula species [43, 44].

3.5. Quercetin (QC)

Quercetin (QC) is found in many plant species as one of the most common flavonoid glycosides. This compound is very useful. Fig. (13) shows its structure. Table 8 presents its NMR data. When UV spectra were recorded after treatment with shift reagents, diagnostic information about its structure was revealed as summarized below.

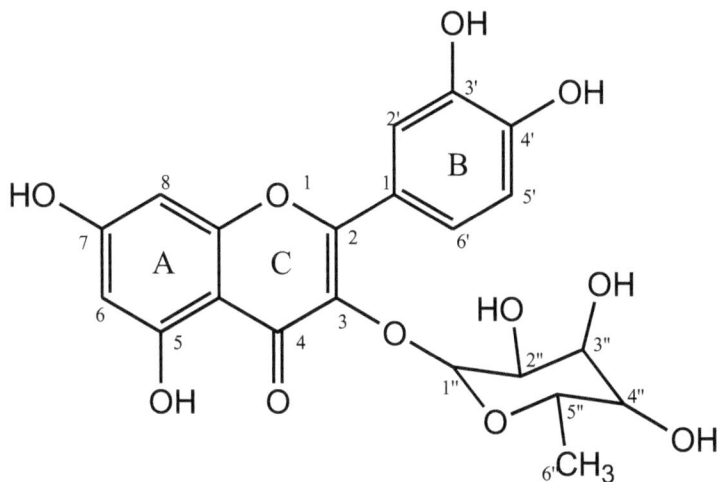

Fig. (13). Chemical structure of compound Quercetin.

Table 8. NMR data of Quercetin.

Proton	H	Carbon	C
2	-	2	156.90 (C)
3	-	3	134.69 (C)
4	-	4	178.20 (C)
4a	-	4a	104.56 (C)
5	-	5	161.75 (C)

Proton	H	Carbon	C
6	6.11 d (2.1)	6	99.15 (CH)
7	-	7	164.63 (C)
8	6.29 d (2.1)	8	94.09 (CH)
8a	-	8a	157.76 (C)
1'	-	1'	121.22 (C)
2'	7.20 d (2.2)	2'	116.13 (CH)
3'	-	3'	145.65 (C)
4'	-	4'	148.88 (C)
5'	6.78 d (9.6)	5'	115.93 (CH)
6'	7.14 dd (9.6, 2.2)	6'	121.58 (CH)
1"	5.15 d (8.1)	1"	102.29 (CH)
2"	4.31	2"	71.03 (CH)
3"	4.57	3"	70.83 (CH)
4"	3.96 brs	4"	71.66 (CH)
5"	4.81	5"	70.51 (CH)
6"	0.73 d (7.1)	6"	17.94 (CH$_3$)

Compound **QC** was eluted with *n*-hexane-ethyl acetate (75:25 *v/v*) of the column and yielded yellow powder, % yield: 0.155% *w/w*; m.p. 175-177 °C

UV (MeOH) λ_{max}: 211, 255, 372 nm (NaOH): 224, 316, 424 nm, (AlCl$_3$): 227, 292, 442 nm, (NaOAc): 223, 314, 402 nm, (NaOAc+H$_3$BO$_3$): 214, 288, 396

IR (KBr) υ_{max}: 3265, 1654, 1502, 1454, 1354 cm^{-1}

FAB-MS *m/z*: 448 [M]$^+$ C$_{21}$H$_{20}$O$_{11}$

CONCLUDING REMARKS

Natural products play an important role in drug discovery, as they act as active principles or act as templates for new drug synthesis. Recent advancements in isolation techniques such as counter-current chromatography, supercritical fluid chromatography, prep-HPLC, and prep-GC provide bioactive and novel natural compounds ready for structural elucidation. Development of hyphenated techniques such as LC-NMR, LC-Mass and GC-MS have drastically hastened natural product isolation and identification. These hyphenated techniques have made simultaneous isolation and identification of natural products possible. The advanced and sophisticated versions of the techniques such as UV-visible, FT-IR,

1D and 2D NMR spectroscopy and mass spectrometry have changed the landscape of phytochemical analysis and structural elucidation of natural products.

ABBREVIATIONS

COSY	Correlation spectroscopy
^{13}C-NMR	^{13}Carbon-NMR
ESI-MS	Electron Spray Ionization mass spectrometry
FT-IR	Fourier transform infrared
GC-MS	Gas chromatography mass spectrometry
HMBC	Heteronuclear multiple-bond coherence
HSQC	Heteronuclear single quantum coherence
^{1}H NMR	Proton NMR
m/z	Mass to charge ratio
LC-Mass	Liquid chromatography mass spectrometry
LC-NMR	Liquid chromatography- Nuclear magnetic resonance
MALDI TOF MS	Matrix-assisted laser desorption/ionization time-of-flight MS
NA	Norgadoleic acid
NMR	Nuclear magnetic resonance
MRM	Multiple reaction monitoring
NOESY	Nuclear overhauser enhancement spectroscopy
OA	Octatriacontenoic acid
SRM	Selected reaction monitoring
TOCSY	Total correlation spectroscopy
UV	Ultra-Violet

CONSENT FOR PUBLICATION

Not applicable.

CONFLICT OF INTEREST

The author(s) confirms that there is no conflict of interest.

ACKNOWLEDGEMENTS

Authors dedicate this chapter to Prof. Mohammad Ali for his contribution to the field of phytochemistry.

REFERENCES

[1] Ali M. Techniques in Terpenoid Identification. Delhi: Birla Publication 2001; pp. 252-61.

[2] Henkel T, Brunne RM, Müller H, Reichel F. Statistical investigation into structural complementarity of natural products and synthetic compounds. Angew Chem Int Ed Engl 1999; 38(5): 643-7.
[http://dx.doi.org/10.1002/(SICI)1521-3773(19990301)38:5<643::AID-ANIE643>3.0.CO;2-G]
[PMID: 29711552]

[3] Balandrin MF, Klocke JA. Medicinal and Aromatic Plants.Springer Verlag. Berlin 1988; pp. 3-36.

[4] Tyler VE, Brady LR, Robert JE. Pharmacognosy, 9th ed, Lea and Febiger, Philadelphia,. 1988.

[5] Kinghorn AD. Phytochemical Resource for Medicine and Agriculture. New York: Plenum 1992; pp. 9-12.

[6] Douglas Kinghorn A. Pharmacognosy in the 21st century. J Pharm Pharmacol 2001; 53(2): 135-48.
[http://dx.doi.org/10.1211/0022357011775334] [PMID: 11273009]

[7] Ali A. Textbook of Pharmacognosy. Delhi: CBS Publisher and Distributors 1997; pp. 14-6.

[8] Ahamad J, Ali M, Mir SR. New Glycoside Esters from the Aerial Parts of *Artemisia absinthium* Linn. Nat Prod J 2013; 3(4): 260-7.
[http://dx.doi.org/10.2174/2210315503041403281113518]

[9] Alkefai NH, Sharma M, Ahamad J, Amin S, Mir SR. New olean-15-ene type gymnemic acids from *Gymnema sylvestre* (Retz.) R.Br. and their antihyperglycemic activity through α-glucosidase inhibition. Phytochem Lett 2019; 32: 83-9.
[http://dx.doi.org/10.1016/j.phytol.2019.05.005]

[10] Ahamad J, Ali M, Mir SR. Isoflavone glycosides from aerial parts of *Artemisia absinthium* Linn. Chem Nat Compd 2014; 49(6): 696-700.
[http://dx.doi.org/10.1007/s10600-014-0807-1]

[11] Hassan N, Ahamad J, Amin S, Mir SR. Rapid preparative isolation of erythrocentaurin from *Enicostemma littorale* by medium pressure liquid chromatography, its estimation by a validated HPTLC densitometric method and α-amylase inhibitory activity. J Sep Sci 2015; 38(4): 592-8.
[http://dx.doi.org/10.1002/jssc.201401030] [PMID: 25504557]

[12] Naquvi KJ, Ali M, Ahmad J. Two new aliphatic lactones from the fruits of *Coriandrum sativum* L. Org Med Chem Lett 2012; 2(1): 28.
[http://dx.doi.org/10.1186/2191-2858-2-28] [PMID: 22800677]

[13] Harborne JB. Phytochemical methods-A guide to modern technique of plant analysis. 3rd ed. London: Chapman and Hall 1998; pp. 109-45.

[14] Trease GE, Evans WC. Pharmacognosy. 16th ed., London: Bailliere Tindall 2009.

[15] Homoeopathic Pharmacopoeia of India, Pharmacopoeia commission for Indian medicine and homoeopathy, Ministry of AYUSH, Government of India, 2019.

[16] Silverstein RM, Webster FX, Kiemle DJ. Spectrometric identification of organic compounds. 7th ed., USA: John Wiley & Sons, Inc 2005.

[17] Alkefai NH, Ahamad J, Amin S, Mir SR. Arylated gymnemic acids from *Gymnema sylvestre* R.Br. as potential α-glucosidase inhibitors. Phytochem Lett 2018; 25: 196-202.
[http://dx.doi.org/10.1016/j.phytol.2018.04.021]

[18] Ahamad J, Ali M, Mir SR. New isoquinoline alkaloids from the stem bark of *Berberis aristata*. Indian J Chem-B 2014; 53: 1237-41.

[19] Bross-Walch N, Kühn T, Moskau D, Zerbe O. Strategies and tools for structure determination of natural products using modern methods of NMR spectroscopy. Chem Biodivers 2005; 2(2): 147-77.
[http://dx.doi.org/10.1002/cbdv.200590000] [PMID: 17191970]

[20] Wishart DS. Characterization of biopharmaceuticals by NMR spectroscopy. Trends Analyt Chem 2013; 48: 96-11.
[http://dx.doi.org/10.1016/j.trac.2013.03.009]

[21] Fukushi E. Advanced NMR approaches for a detailed structure analysis of natural products. Biosci Biotechnol Biochem 2006; 70(8): 1803-12.
[http://dx.doi.org/10.1271/bbb.50663] [PMID: 16926490]

[22] Reynolds WF, Mazzola EP. Nuclear magnetic resonance in the structural elucidation of natural products.Progress in the chemistry of organic natural products, Methodology. Heidelberg: Springer 2015; pp. 223-310.
[http://dx.doi.org/10.1007/978-3-319-05275-5_3]

[23] Breton RC, Reynolds WF. Using NMR to identify and characterize natural products. Nat Prod Rep 2013; 30(4): 501-24.
[http://dx.doi.org/10.1039/c2np20104f] [PMID: 23291908]

[24] Martin GE. Using 1,1- and 1,n-ADEQUATE 2D NMR data in structure elucidation protocols. Annu Rep NMR Spectrosc 2011; 74: 215-91.
[http://dx.doi.org/10.1016/B978-0-08-097072-1.00005-4]

[25] Naquvi KJ, Ali M, Ahamad J. Two new phytosterols from the stem bark of *Ficus bengalensis* L. J Saudi Chem Soc 2015; 19: 650-4.
[http://dx.doi.org/10.1016/j.jscs.2012.06.006]

[26] Ali M, Naquvi KJ, Ahamad J, Mir SR. Three new esters from the stem bark of *Ficus bengalensis*. J Pharm Res 2010; 3(2): 352-5.

[27] Johnson D, Orlando R. Optimization of data-dependent parameters for LC-MS/MS protein identification. J Biomol Tech 2011; 22 (Suppl.): S57-8.

[28] Shevchenko A, Jensen ON, Podtelejnikov AV, *et al.* Linking genome and proteome by mass spectrometry: large-scale identification of yeast proteins from two dimensional gels. Proc Natl Acad Sci USA 1996; 93(25): 14440-5.
[http://dx.doi.org/10.1073/pnas.93.25.14440] [PMID: 8962070]

[29] Matros A, Kaspar S, Witzel K, Mock HP. Recent progress in liquid chromatography-based separation and label-free quantitative plant proteomics. Phytochemistry 2011; 72(10): 963-74.
[http://dx.doi.org/10.1016/j.phytochem.2010.11.009] [PMID: 21176926]

[30] Delahunty C, Yates JR III. Protein identification using 2D-LC-MS/MS. Methods 2005; 35(3): 248-55.
[http://dx.doi.org/10.1016/j.ymeth.2004.08.016] [PMID: 15722221]

[31] Washburn MP, Ulaszek R, Deciu C, Schieltz DM, Yates JR III. Analysis of quantitative proteomic data generated via multidimensional protein identification technology. Anal Chem 2002; 74(7): 1650-7.
[http://dx.doi.org/10.1021/ac015704l] [PMID: 12043600]

[32] Wolters DA, Washburn MP, Yates JR III. An automated multidimensional protein identification technology for shotgun proteomics. Anal Chem 2001; 73(23): 5683-90.
[http://dx.doi.org/10.1021/ac010617e] [PMID: 11774908]

[33] Gilar M, Olivova P, Daly AE, Gebler JC. Two-dimensional separation of peptides using RP-RP-HPLC system with different pH in first and second separation dimensions. J Sep Sci 2005; 28(14): 1694-703.
[http://dx.doi.org/10.1002/jssc.200500116] [PMID: 16224963]

[34] Thomas R. Spectroscopy (Spectroscopy Tutorial) 2001; 16: 28-37.https://www.spectroscopy-online.com/

[35] Rauh M. LC-MS/MS for protein and peptide quantification in clinical chemistry. J Chromatogr B Analyt Technol Biomed Life Sci 2012; 883-884: 59-67.
[http://dx.doi.org/10.1016/j.jchromb.2011.09.030] [PMID: 22000960]

[36]   Bhushan D, Pandey A, Choudhary MK, Datta A, Chakraborty S, Chakraborty N. Comparative proteomics analysis of differentially expressed proteins in chickpea extracellular matrix during dehydration stress. Mol Cell Proteomics 2007; 6(11): 1868-84.
[http://dx.doi.org/10.1074/mcp.M700015-MCP200] [PMID: 17686759]

[37]   Peiren N, Vanrobaeys F, de Graaf DC, Devreese B, Van Beeumen J, Jacobs FJ. The protein composition of honeybee venom reconsidered by a proteomic approach. Biochim Biophys Acta 2005; 1752(1): 1-5.
[http://dx.doi.org/10.1016/j.bbapap.2005.07.017] [PMID: 16112630]

[38]   Schmelzer CE, Schöps R, Ulbrich-Hofmann R, Neubert RH, Raith K. Mass spectrometric characterization of peptides derived by peptic cleavage of bovine β-casein. J Chromatogr A 2004; 1055(1-2): 87-92.
[http://dx.doi.org/10.1016/j.chroma.2004.09.003] [PMID: 15560483]

[39]   Matysiak J, Schmelzer CEH, Neubert RHH, Kokot ZJ. Characterization of honeybee venom by MALDI-TOF and nanoESI-QqTOF mass spectrometry. J Pharm Biomed Anal 2011; 54(2): 273-8.
[http://dx.doi.org/10.1016/j.jpba.2010.08.020] [PMID: 20850943]

[40]   Gonnet F, Lemaître G, Waksman G, Tortajada J. MALDI/MS peptide mass fingerprinting for proteome analysis: identification of hydrophobic proteins attached to eucaryote keratinocyte cytoplasmic membrane using different matrices in concert. Proteome Sci 2003; 1(1): 2.
[http://dx.doi.org/10.1186/1477-5956-1-2] [PMID: 12769822]

[41]   Blonder J, Conrads TP, Veenstra TD. Characterization and quantitation of membrane proteomes using multidimensional MS-based proteomic technologies. Expert Rev Proteomics 2004; 1(2): 153-63.
[http://dx.doi.org/10.1586/14789450.1.2.153] [PMID: 15966810]

[42]   Fortin T, Salvador A, Charrier JP, *et al.* Multiple reaction monitoring cubed for protein quantification at the low nanogram/milliliter level in nondepleted human serum. Anal Chem 2009; 81(22): 9343-52.
[http://dx.doi.org/10.1021/ac901447h] [PMID: 19839594]

[43]   Seca AML, Pinto DCGA, Silva AMS. Metabolomic profile of the genus *Inula*. Chem Biodivers 2015; 12(6): 859-906.
[http://dx.doi.org/10.1002/cbdv.201400080] [PMID: 26080736]

[44]   Zhang B, Zeng J, Yan Y, *et al.* Ethyl acetate extract from *Inula helenium L.* inhibits the proliferation of pancreatic cancer cells by regulating the STAT3/AKT pathway. Mol Med Rep 2018; 17(4): 5440-8.
[PMID: 29393456]

CHAPTER 6

Pharmacological Evaluation of Herbal Medicine

Subasini Uthirapathy[1,*], Javed Ahamad[2], Jaswanth Albert[3] and **Govind Prasad Dubey[4,*]**

[1] *Department of Pharmacology, Faculty of Pharmacy, Tishk International University, KRG, Iraq*

[2] *Department of Pharmacognosy, Faculty of Pharmacy, Tishk International University, KRG, Iraq*

[3] *Faculty of Pharmacology, Surabhi Dayakar Rao College of Pharmacy, Gajwel, Rimmanaguda, Hyderabad, Telangana, India*

[4] *Institute of Medical Sciences, Banaras Hindu University, Varanasi, India*

Abstract: Natural products broadly incorporate plant-based product as well as marine, plants, microorganisms and minerals. There are several animal products that are also consumed by humans as a food health supplement and also medicine. Herbal products have a variety of phytocompounds. . The identification of these molecules is essential for standardization and quality control of the herbal products. The world wide variety of plants and their species have been identified and *i.e.* 250000. Morphological and chemical constituents of plant species vary from one ethnic group to another. Humidity, temperature and altitude soil conditions are all responsible for both structural and functional characteristics of the natural products. Therefore standardization and quality control are the big challenges before using natural products. Heavy metal toxicity, microbial load and aflotoxin are the major and important parameters of evaluation of the safety profile of the natural products. Therefore, before using the natural product, we should characterized the structural variation to establish structural and functional relationships. In the present paper, some of the experimental models have been described, which will be useful in the preparation of standard plant based products.In order to provide standard product, some important experimental methods have been described in this paper. Herbal medicinal products have a wide scope of assorted variety of multidimensional synthetic structures; in the ongoing occasions, the utility of normal items as natural capacity modifiers has impressive consideration. The botanical study evaluated the identification of 250,000 to 350,000 plant species over the planet. Notwithstanding, only around 35,000 species have been utilized in various networks of the world for the treatment of different infirmities. Nonetheless, this exceptional fortune needs exhaustive consideration as far as biological and pharmacological screening to serve humankind against different diseases. The traditional system of treatment, varying in idea and convention, represents well-created frameworks, for example, Allopathic, Homeopathic, Ayurvedic

* **Corresponding author Dr. Govind Prasad Dubey and Subasini Uthirapathy:** Institute of Medical Sciences, Banaras Hindu University, Varanasi, India; Tel: +0091 9450 9639 42 and Department of Pharmacology, Faculty of Pharmacy, Tishk International University, KRG, Iraq; E-mails: gpdubey13@gmail.com & subasini.uthirapathy@tiu.edu.iq

and Chinese system of treatment. A large portion of the enlightened countries has built up their own *Materia Medica*, assembling insights concerning different plants utilized for remedial purposes. This chapteris focused on the diverse pharmacological screening techniques with point by point illustration of genuine biological investigations that are useful to discover new bioactive phytochemicals in antidiabetic, analgesic,anti-inflammatory, neuroprotective, anti-obesity, and depression disorders and so on. Preclinical study is strictly required to follow CPCSEA guideline into the pharmacological practical.This chapter provides essential knowledge of practical features of the experimental Screening pharmacology right from laboratory animal handling, the important techniques and methodology used in experimental pharmacology. The experimental procedure described in this chapter is planned on the basis of strong technical materials and personal knowledge in hands-on experiments under the guidance of renowned personalities. This chapter is arranged to understand the experimental animal handling techniques by witnessing the induction experiments. These experimental procedures will be helpful for graduates and postgraduates students associated with pharmacology, toxicology and researcher. Simple and newer animal models have been combined, which may help the students to occupy in new drug development activities. Also, some important points have been conferred *e.g.* ethics of animal experimentation, blood collection techniques, euthanasia, animal care and handling.

Keywords: Anti-inflammatory Activity, Antidiabetic Activity, Anti-Obesity, Bio-Logical Approach, Drug Discovery, Herbal Medicinal Products, Neuropharmacology, Pharmacological Evaluation.

1. INTRODUCTION

Standardization of natural products is complex and challenging. It requires a multidisciplinary approach to prove the therapeutic value of plant-based medicine in comparison to synthetic chemicals. Plant-based natural products are used for the centuries. The traditional knowledge which is a practice in the form of Ayurveda, Siddha, Unani and Chinese medicine. Generally, the traditional form of medicine utilizes multiple herbs so poly-herbal and poly-molecular formulation require providing pharmacological action, bioavailability and bioequivalence study to compare the risk-benefit ratio in comparison to synthetic chemicals. The approach of the above system of traditional medicine is holistic. Therefore, to meet the national and international regulatory norms, several guidelines have been framed by different countries. The universal acceptance of traditional medicine requires-complying regulatory norms. In the present book chapter, we have described the experimental model required in the including toxico-kinetic and toxicodynamic effect to provide the scientific basis of natural products. Medication discovery is prompting to be a challenging logical undertaking to discover strong and suitable lead applicants, which is only the procedure stream from a screening of regular items to another disengage that requires ability and experience. It portrays the bioactive compounds obtained from natural resources, its phytochemical examination, characterization and pharmacological examination. The trial on animals gives a general thought regarding the tested medication (pharmacodynamics, pharmacokinetic and toxicology) through different strategies engaged with the procedure. In any case, a definitive objective of any medication research is to utilize the medication in the patient's care [1]. The preclinical study is principally intended to discover a lead compound with wanting adequacy and well-being for clinical study through pharmacokinetics and pharmacodynamics information acquired from *in vitro* and *in vivo* investigations. Pharmacology is a therapeutic science that structures a spine of the restorative calling as medications structure the foundation of treatment in human ailments. Consequently, it is of most extreme significance to portray the pharmacological basis of therapeutics to expand the advantages and limit the dangers of medications to beneficiaries [2].

Broadly experimental animals are divided into three categories such as Rodents (Mouse, Rat, Guinea pig, black mice, Hamster *etc.*), non-Rodents (Rabbit, Dog, Cat, Monkey, Pig *etc.*) and miscellaneous (Frog, Pigeon, Zebrafish, Chicken). The proper selection of animal models is one of the paramount steps in the evaluation of new drugs pharmacologically.The animal model preferred for the study must be producing a similar disease profile as in the human. Once preclinical is approved, it can be conducted under CPCSEA (Committee for the Purpose of Control and Supervision of Experiments in Animals) guidelines.Bioassays are designed to check the pharmacological activity or efficacy of a new drug, to find the role of endogenous ligands and to find drug toxicity [3]. This book chapter note on pharmacology is principally a note for undergraduate wellbeing science students, for example, wellbeing official, nursing, birthing assistance and lab innovation students. In any case, other wellbeing experts whose career includes drug treatment or related viewpoints ought to likewise discover a significant part of the material applicable. The objective of this book chapter is to find out the therapeutic effect; to study the toxicity, and; to study the mechanism and site of action of drugs. Bioassay is the process of evaluation of the drug biologically. In this chapter, we discussed common laboratory animals used pharmacological screening, ethics of animal experimentation, and pharmacological screening methods of major human diseases.

2. COMMON LABORATORY ANIMALS

2.1. Albino Rats (*Rattus Norvegicus*)

Two strains were commonly used: (a)Wistar Rats and (b) Sprague Dawley Rats. The normal weight of these rats ranges from 150-300g. The main advantages of Albino Rats are: docile and small in size, easy to handle, a drug to be tested is required in only small quantities.

2.2. Albino Mice (*Mus musculus*)

These are the smallest laboratory animals and a common strain is Swiss albino mice. The normal weight ranges from 20-30g.The main uses of these animals are: highly docile, maintain expenses are less, sensitive to a very small quantity of drug and it is mainly used for screening of anti-cancer drugs, endocrine disorder, and immunological diseases.

2.3. C57BL/6 (B6) Black Mice

It is a common inbred strain of laboratory mouse. It is the most widely used "genetic background" for genetically modified mice for use as models of human disease. This mouse has a dark brown to black. They are more sensitive to noise and odors.

2.4. Guinea Pigs (*Cavia porcellus*)

These are highly docile and easy to handle, highly sensitive to histamine, they are not able to synthesize required vitamin- C and it is supplied exogenously. These animals are mainly used for: bioassay of histamine and digitalis, and arethe ideal models for anaphylactic shock.

2.5. Rabbits (*Lupas cuniculus*)

These are white strains from New Zealand and are widely used.They have huge caseum and long appendix, and they contain enzyme atropine esterase in the liver and plasma so they can tolerate a high dose of atropine. These are mainly used for pyrogen testing and ideal for pharmacokinetics studies.

3. ETHICS OF ANIMAL EXPERIMENTATION

3.1. Objectives of Anesthesia

Eliminate or minimize the potential procedures that may cause the animal pain, distress or discomfort.

3.2. Pre-Anesthetic Medications

To achieve satisfactory anesthesia and to minimize the anesthesia complications.

The following drugs were administered before surgery or during pharmacological evaluation:

Anti cholinergics - reduces bronchial & salivary secretion

Sedatives - reduces fear and stress

α_2-Adrenergic agonist - moderate analgesic

Opioids - analgesic, decrease anxiety

Anti-emetics - decrease post-operative vomiting

H_2-Blockers - prevent ulcer

Benzodiazepines - reduce the excitation

3.3. Drugs

Table 1. The following drugs were administered before surgery or during pharmacological evaluation.

DRUG	MOUSE	RAT	GUINEA PIG	RABBIT
Ketamine	✓	✓	✓	✓
Phenobarbitone	✓	✓	✓	✓
Thiopentone	✓	✓	✓	-
Isoflurane	✓	✓	✓	✓
Enflurane	✓	✓	✓	✓
α-chloralose	-	-	-	✓
Ketamine+xylazine	✓	✓	✓	✓
Ketamine+diazepam	-	✓	✓	-
Ketamine+medatomidine	✓	✓	✓	✓

3.4. Standard Bleeding Techniques [3]

Blood samples are regularly collected from experimental animals to study the effect of the drug on biochemical parameters. Blood collection is carried out in conscious animals. The animal's tail is dipped by the xylol or warm water to increase the circulations of blood in the tail. The needle is inserted into the tail; the blood is slowly aspirated without damage the tail of the vein. Blood collection used a needle reduces the impurity of the sample. The sampling procedures for blood collection are of two types.

A. Blood collection without mortality (survival bleeding)
B. Blood collection with mortality (non-survival bleeding)

Phlebotomist: People who are trained to draw blood by vein puncture.

Blood collection without mortality:

A. Tail vein

B. Saphenous vein

C. Jugular vein

D. Retro-orbital vein

E. Marginal ear vein

Blood collection with mortality:

A. Cardiac puncture

B. Arterial cannulation

Factors to be considered in blood collection: following factors should be considered during blood collection:

A. The species going to be used

B. Size of the animal and total blood volume

C. Amount of blood required

D. The frequency of sampling

E. The effect of anesthesia on blood going to measure

F. Training and experience of the phlebotomist.

3.5. Euthanasia

Euthanasia is the humane allowing dying animals. The animals are quickly renderedthem unconscious and subsequent death without stress and pain. The method of euthanasia depends upon the species of animals and restraint methods. It is very important that, in an experimental setting, the method of euthanasia must be primarily consistent with the experimental goals. Whenever an animal is killed in research teaching and testing, it must be done with safety and emotional effect, reliability, and irreversibility and in a way that ensures the death contain as possibly as minimum pain, distress and anxiety [3, 4].

Recognitions and confirmations of death:

A. Cessation of respiration of heartbeat and absence of reflexes are good indications of irreversible death in rodents

B. Death may be confirmed by excogitation or extraction of the heart, the evisceration of deep freezing and decapitation.

3.6. Types of Euthanasia

3.6.1. Physical Methods

Physical methods of killing rodents, deliberation must be assumed to careful management and restraint of the animal before the killing, cervical dislocation, decapitation, capitative bolt, concussion, electrical stunning, rapid freezing, and microwave.

Cervical dislocation: It's the breaking of the backbone near the head. It causes extensive damage to the brain stem resulting in immediate unconsciousness and death.

Decapitation: The immediate lack of blood circulation to the heart and brain and subsequent anoxia is thought to the head shuts down.

Capitative Bolt: This method is used for larger size animals like rabbits. Capitative bolts designed specifically penetrate about 3cm into the brain.

Concussion: This involves a blow to the back of the head and causes damage to the brain and the animal becomes inert.

Electrical Stunning: In this method a current pass directly to the brain and ensure immediate unconsciousness.

Rapid freezing: This method placing the animal in liquid nitrogen, only fetus and neonates were killed by this method.

Microwave: This method is not commonly used for euthanasia. It involves a specialized apparatus [4].

3.6.1.1. Chemical Methods

An increase in the concentration of anesthetics will lead to respiratory depression and finally death. This method is most commonly used to induce euthanasia. Volatile inhalational anesthetics like chloroform, ether, *etc.* and injectable agents such as sodium pentobarbitone, and ketamine are also used. Ethanol (70%) was administered intra-peritoneally but it will produce irritation hence it is used only with unconscious animals [4]. Carbon dioxide (CO_2) is presently considered to be a safe and humane method of euthanasia that has been ideal technique for animals. The CO_2 is inexpensive, non-flammable and non-explosive. The use of a proper chamber permits a group of animals to be speedily euthanized simultaneously.

3. PHARMACOLOGICAL EVALUATION METHODS

3.1. Evaluation of Analgesic Activity of Herbal Medicine

3.1.1. Hotplate Analgesiometer Method

The method deals withthe principle of the thermal radiation heat. This principle is used in the animal experiment for the evaluation of the centrally acting analgesics, and hence this method is found to be the differentiating factor between the centrally acting opiates and non-opiates analgesics. The screening of central analgesic activity can be performed by using Eddy's hot plate apparatus [5]. The instrument involved is known as "hotplate analgesiometer". The instrument consists of an electrically heated surface (made up of iron, aluminum or copper) whose temperature is maintained by the thermostat 'Knob' at 55°C to 56 °C.The animals are placed on a hot plate; the animal shows such a response in 5-6 seconds. The control group is given 1% acacia orally while the standard group was treated with Pentazocin (6 mg/kg b.wt.) intra-peritoneally. After maintaining the temperature mouse /rat are placed on the hot plate and observed for either paw licking or jumping reaction. The reaction time is recorded by a stop-watch. Repeated reading is taken at 20, 60, and 90 minutes after the drug administration. Cut off time for a rat is 20-30 sec and for mice, it is 15-20 sec.

3.1.2. Tail Clip Method

Analgesia is characterized as a condition of diminished attention to pain and analgesics are substances thatstop pain sensation. The common analgesics are paracetamol, aspirin and morphine. The painful reactions in animals can be delivered by applying noxious(unpleasant) stimulation for example, (1) increasing the temperature (2) using synthetic compounds (acidic corrosive, bradykinin), (3) inducing physical pressure (tail immersion) in the research center. For physical pressure, an artery clip is placed on the tip of the tail in mice to induce pain. The animal response to noxious stimuli by biting the clip or try to remove the clip is taken as the reaction time takes to 2 or 3 basal reaction times. Pentazocine is used as a standard drug to note the response time at 15 mininterval upto 1 hr (cutoff time is 15sec). Compute the rate expanding response time (record of pain-relieving movement) [6, 7].

3.1.3. Tail Flick Method

The tail flick method is used for assessing the analgesic activity of herbal medicinal products. In this method, we measure the threshold response at which rat/ mice escape tails. In this method,a wire which warmed upto 55 °C is utilized and radiant heat is applied. For this purpose, analgesiometer is used. Animals are screened on apparatus and cut off time is recorded after > 5 seconds [6, 7].The percentage of antinociception is calculated by the following equation.

$$\text{Antinociception (\%)} = \frac{\text{Test latency} - \text{Control latency}}{\text{Cut off time} - \text{Control latency}} \times 100$$

3.1.4. Acetic Acid-Induced Writhing

The painful reaction in experimental animals can be produced by acetic acid. Intra-peritoneal injection of acetic acid produces a pain reaction, which is characterized as withdrawing of the limb, stretching of the body, retraction of the abdomen and stomach touches the ground are taken as writhing response. Analgesics, both narcotics and non-narcotic types, inhibit writhing response. These experimental models of pain are commonly used to test response thresholds to high-intensity stimuli (acute pain tests) or persistent pain models. The tail-flick test is predominantly a spinal response while hot-plate is mostly at the supraspinal level [8].

3.2. Evaluation of Anti-Inflammatory Activity of Herbal Medicine

The herbal medicinal products regularly evaluated for their anti-inflammatory activity using carrageenan-induced paw edema method. The principle of screening of anti-inflammatory agents is based on the reduction of edema caused by any irritant or phlogistic agent (the agent that may induce inflammation or fever). The edema is measured by an instrument known as Plethysmograph.The rat paw is immersed into the tube 'A' and the reading is checked through the tube 'B' (some set-up has a digital display attached to it). Plethysmographis the apparatus used to measure of the paw volume the changes in volume. In the experiment, it measures the volume of the rat paw in the presence and absence of irritant and after the treatment of anti-inflammatory drugs (Fig. **1**).The rats are divided into 2 groups (n = 6). The test groups are treated with indomethacin (8 mg/kg, p.o.) and control groups' saline peroral and the paw volume is measured at 30, 60, 120, and 180 min after carrageenan using a Plethysmometer [9 - 11]. The animals are pretreated with the test drug 1 h before the administration of carrageenan (Fig. **1**). Acute inflammation was formed by the sub-planter administration of 0.1 ml of (1%, w/v) carrageenan in normal saline in the right paw of the rats. The left paw will serve as a non-flamed paw for comparisons. Calculate the percentage difference in the right and left paw volume of each rat of the control and test group.

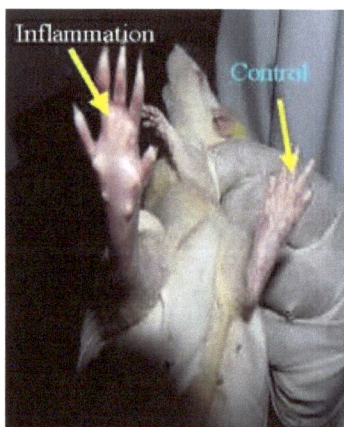

Fig. (1). Carrageenan-induced paw edema.

Anti-inflammatory activity (%) = (1-T)/C×100

Where T represents the percentages of difference in paw volume before and after test drugs. C represents the percentages of the difference of volume in the control groups.

3.3. Evaluation of Pupil Size Effects of Herbal Medicine

Miotics (constrict the pupil) and mydriatics drugs (dilate the pupils) are generally screened by this method. The role of circular muscle, radial muscle and ciliary muscle is well-known. The eye is supplied with both the sympathetic and parasympathetic nervous system. The pupil diameter is controlled by radial muscle and circular muscle. Radial muscle is innervated with sympathetic nerves and circular muscle with parasympathetic nerves. When the anticholinergic drugs/para-sympatholytic is instilled in the eye, it blocks the M_3-receptor. It leads to paralysis of circular muscle and dilates the pupil which turns increases the pupil size. The conduction is termed as mydriasis [12]. Keep the rabbit inconvenient position that the head will be extended outside. Consider its right eye as control (2-3 drops of saline are instilled in this eye) and left eye as the test eye (2-3 drops of test drug is instilled in this eye). At that point, we need to test reflexes. Corneal touch reflexes study by touching the cornea of the eye with cotton buds and seeing whether the rabbit blinking the eyelids or not. Check both the control eye and test eye. Light reflexes by concentrating a torchlight on the eye and observing whether the pupil is tightened (constricted) because of light or not. The effect of test drug on the diameter of pupils are observed by the dilation or constriction of the pupil after adding the test solution is observed and compared with the diameter of pupil in both eyes.

3.4. Evaluation of the Hypnotic Effect of Herbal Medicine

Hypnosis is the process of natural sleep and the drugs or agents inducing it are known as the hypnotic agents. This concept applies to the patient or human use, but in the animal experiments, the term "hypnotic" means central depression which induces unconsciousness, associated with loss of righting reflexes and muscle relaxation. The "loss of righting reflex" is the term mainly used to denote the 'sleep' of an animal and it is defined as the loss of postural reaction which can't be corrected when the animal is kept on its back. In the righting reflex, animal turns body in such a way that, its paws or feet are pointed at the ground. The righting reflex reaction is dependent on normal vestibular, visual and proprioceptive functions.The righting reflex is the ability of the animal to maintain posture or position [13, 14]. First, choose mice/rats divided into three groups. The first group receives 0.1ml of saline in the i.p. route. The second group gets diazepam (5mg/kg i.p) and the third group received test drug, the volume of the drug injected should not exceed 0.5 ml in mice. The time of the onset of action is the loss of righting reflex in mice *i.e.* the mice neglects to maintain its normal posture or falls asleep (hypnosis) is recorded for each animal. The animals are put on the table, leaving sufficient space. The time of recovery from sleep is recorded.

It is the time from the loss of righting reflex and the time when the animal turns to recover its normal position [16].

3.5. Evaluation of Muscle Relaxant Activity of Herbal Medicine

A muscle relaxant is a drug which affects the skeletal muscle functions and decreases the muscle tone. It is used to reduce muscle spasms, pain and hyper-reflexes. Diazepam is a class of CNS depressant also has muscle relaxant activity along with sedative and hypnotics. The loss of pain grip is an indication of muscle relaxation. Rotarod test is used to evaluate the fore and hind limb motor coordination of rodents. The apparatus consists of a horizontal metal rod (coated with rubber) of 3 cm diameter attached to a motor with speed adjusted to 2-6 rotations/min. The cut off time for the test is 2 min. The retention time for each mouse/rat is recorded in seconds [15, 16].

3.6. Evaluation Of Anti-Anxiety Effect Of Herbal Medicine

It is a method for the selective identification of the anxiolytic effect of drugs in rodents. The elevated plus-maze apparatus having two open arms and two closed arms and an open roof of the entire maze elevated from the floor. The animals are placed individually at the center of the elevated plus-maze with their head facing towards the open arm during the 1.5-5 min test. Rat or mice is allowed to explore the maze for about 5 min. When animals are treated with the anti-anxiety drugs, the number of animal (rat or mice) entries to closed arm became much closer or equal to open arm. The no. of entries in closed arms reflects the relative safety and no. of entries in open arms reflects the relative fearfulness. Normally mice or rat natural avoidance of open space, feels safe in dark space and prefers closed-arm first. Anxiolytic drugs are expected equal to open or close arm that means the number of entries and the number of times spent equal to open/close arm [15, 16].

3.7. Evaluation of Local Anesthetic Activity of Herbal Medicine

Local anesthetics are agents which block conduction of Na^+ by decreasing or preventing the large transient increase in the permeability of excitable membranes and at higher concentration, they also block K^+ channels. This is the basic principle for loss of the sensation, even after givenan external stimulus [17].

3.8. Evaluation of Anti-Peptic-Ulcer Activity of Herbal Medicine

3.8.1. Ethanol-Induced Ulcer Model

Animals are divided into five groups of six animals in each group. Group 1 animals served as a vehicle control group. They received only a vehicle equivalent to the volume of the test drug. Group 2 animals are represented as a diseased control group. Ulceration is produced by the administration of absolute alcohol (1 ml to each /rat) orally. Group 3 animals are assigned as the standard drug treatment groups. They received omeprazole (30 mg/kg) by intraperitoneal route. One hour after the treatment of standard drugs, animals are administrated with 1 ml of absolute alcohol orally. Group 4 animals are allocated as test drugs low dose treatment group by intraperitoneal route. One hour after the treatment of low dose test drugs, animals are administrated with 1 ml of absolute alcohol orally. Group 5 animals are allotted as test drug high dose treatment group by intraperitoneal route. One hour after the treatment of high dose test drugs, animals are administrated with 1 ml of absolute alcohol orally. The following parameters will be analyzed such as the total area of the stomach, total glandular area, total ulcerated area, ulcer index, percentage protective index, gross pathology, histopathology [17].

3.8.2. Pylorus Ligation Method (Shay Method)

The animal is anesthetized and a midline abdominal incision is made. The stomach is identified and the pylorus is ligated operatively. Then, leave the animal in the individual cages for 19-24 hr. The test compounds are given either orally (gavage) or injected subcutaneously 30 min before ligation. At a specified time, the animal is sacrificed under euthanasia. The abdomen is opened and a first ligature is placed around the esophagus close to the diaphragm to stop the contents in the stomach. Then, the stomach is removed, and the contents are drained in a centrifuge tube. The volume of the gastric content is measured and then, after, centrifugation, acidity is determined by titration with 0.1N NaOH.

3.8.3. Indomethacin Induced Ulcer

The test drugs dissolved in 0.1% Tween 80 solution are administered orally 10 min before indomethacin (dose 20 mg/kg per oral) which is dissolved in 0.1% Tween 80 solution. After six hours, the rats are killed by anesthesia, and the stomach is removed [17 - 19].

3.8.4. Assessment of Gastric Mucosal Lesions

One hour after alcohol administration rats are sacrificed by an overdose of ether. Their stomachs are removed and opened along the greater curvature. Then, they are washed with ice-cold phosphate-buffered saline (PBS) and scored for macroscopic gross mucosal lesions.The area of hemorrhagic ulcer and petechiation in the glandular part of the stomach is traced on the transparency graph sheet. After that, the stomachs are fixed in 10% buffered formalin solution for histopathological study [20]. Ulcer index (UI) is calculated by the formula:

$$\text{Ulcer Index} = 10 \, / \, X$$

where X = total mucosal area of the glandular part of the stomach/total ulcerated area.

The protective index (PI) of a drug was calculated from the following equation:

$$\text{Protective index (PI)} = \frac{\text{UI of diseased group} - \text{UI of treated group}}{\text{UI of diseased group}} \times 100$$

3.9. Evaluation of Anti-Depressant Effect of Herbal Medicine

Depression includes diminished confidence inthe person. It is normally brought about by response to some exogenous stimuli or might be because of an endogenous emotional reason. In this technique, mice are placed in a glass container containing water. The components of the glass containers can be 40 cm height and 18 cm diameter. Water can be upto 15 cm. This is a reason-ablyinexpensive method; you need not purchase any costly instrument. Animals are prepared for swimming for 15 minutes. Mice when left in the water start swimming. When despondency sets in, they quit swimming. This is considered a fixed status period. In this period mouse does exertion just to keep the head over the water. There is no dynamic swimming. The test is led 24 hours after training. After training 8 animals are chosen for this investigation. There are partitioned into 2 gatherings. Group 4, animals are given ordinary saline (group A) by intraperitoneal route (i.p.), and another groupisgiven test drug (for example imipramine 10mg/kg i.p., group B). The total immovability period is noted for every mouse [20, 21].

Name and sources of herbal drugs: *Epimedium brevicornum, Chrystactinia Mexicana, Chamaemelun nobile, Magnolis officinalis, Hypercum perforatum Lavandula officinalis, Radix Angelicae sinensis, Poria cocos, Rhizoma Alisma orientalis, Radix Paeonia lactiflora,* and *Rhizoma Ligusticumchuanxiong etc.,* These herbal plants have been described to utilize ideal pharmacological effects in treating depression in different animal models.

Preparations: The dried plant is extracted with n-hexane at room temperature for 15-20 days. Thereafter, the extract is filtered and then concentrated under reduced pressure. The maceration process is repeated three times. These above herbal plants and bioactive molecules derived from these plants have exposed antidepressant properties [37 - 40].

3.10. Evaluation of Anti-AtherosclerosisActivity of Herbal Medicine

For evaluation of anti-atherosclerosis activity generally, male rabbits of 8-10 weeks of age are selected. For evaluation of anti-atherosclerosis activity total cholesterol, total glycerides and blood sugar levels are assessed.The rabbit's feeds are changed from commercial food to cholesterol (2%) rich dietand kept on this routine for a time of 10-12 weeks. Rabbits are divided into two groups. One groupis kept on a normal diet and other groups are kept on a cholesterol diet. Atthe end of the experiment, blood is collected for investigation.The animals are sacrificed and the thoracic aorta is evacuated, cleaned of encompassing tissues, and longitudinally cut and opened for an obsession with formaldehyde. The tissue is re-colored with oil red. In animals fed with a normal diet; the aorta doesn't demonstrate any re-coloring, though in cholesterol-fed rabbits the aorta indicates extreme atherogenic sores [22 - 24].

Hyperlipidemia is induced by a diet rich in cholesterol. The anti-atherogenic effect of the drug is studied in diabetic rats induced by Streptozotocin. The effect of the drug is also analyzed in alcohol and nicotine-induced atherogenesis.The efficacy of the test formulation is also studied in the isoproterenol-induced myocardial infarction model. Various respiratory enzymes, antioxidant enzymes and other diagnostic enzymes such as SGOT, SGPT, CPK, and CK (MB) are analyzed.

Recently, it has been identified that high levels of homocysteine, apolipoproteins in the blood are one of the risk factors of atherogenesis. Hence, the role of homocysteine and apolipoproteins are also studied using the test formulation.In all the above experimental inductions, the efficacy of the drug formulation is validated and its mode of action is studied by analyzing the following parameters. Total cholesterol, triglycerides, HDL, LDL, phospholipids Apo A, Apo B, Lp (a), homocysteine, protein, glucose, calcium, electrolytes such as sodium, potassium and chlorides, antioxidants such as vitamin A, E and C.The various lipo-metabolizing enzymes such as lipoprotein lipase, hepatic lipase, LCAT, HMG-CoA reductase, protein kinase, antioxidant enzymes such as SOD, catalase, glutathione peroxidase, glutathione reductase and other enzymes such as SGOT,

SGPT, LDH, CPK, CK (MB) and the respiratory cycle enzymes are assayed. Further, the immunological parameters that influence atherosclerosis, namely cytokines and interleukins are measured [2, 4, 23 - 26].

Name of sources and preparations: *Tribulus terrestris* extract, an aqueous extract of *Ocimum basilicum,* ethanol extract of *Terminalia arjuna*, polysaccharids from *Polygonatum sibiricum*, sweritamarin from *Encostemma littorale, Hypericum perfortum* extract, flowers of *Nelumbo nucifera*, propolis, thymoquinone from *Nigella sativa*. Plant-based bioactive molecules including flavonoids, phenols, tannins and saponins, macro-micro nutrients and antioxidants can be effective atherosclerosis and associated diseases [41, 42].

3.11. Evaluation of Anti-diabetic Activity of Herbal Medicine

For the screening of anti-diabetic drugs several *in-vitro* and animal models have been reported which include chemical, surgical and genetic models. The selection of appropriate animal models has been identified as one of the common problems associated with the success of drug discovery. For the *in-vitro* evaluation α-amylase and α-glucosidase enzyme inhibition assay are used. For chemical induction of diabetes mellitus, alloxan and streptozotocin are regularly used in animal models. Streptozotocin (STZ) is considered as a better agent for the induction of diabetes in animal models. Weigh the animals and number them and calculate the dose. The collection of the blood from pretreated animals by retro-orbital sinus and plasma glucose level is measured. Administration of drug (saline, std and test drug) by orally for all groups once a day from 1-28 days. The rats are fasted for 16 hr before the induction of diabetes *via* intraperitoneal route injection of streptozotocin (STZ 55 mg/kg) in 0.1 M cold citrate buffer (pH 4.5) by IP route for all the group of animals. The remaining rats, representing the non-diabetic group, are injected with buffer alone. The STZ administered rats are permissible to drink 5% glucose solution dramatic to overwhelm the drug-induced hyperglycemia. Hyperglycaemia is confirmed after induction *via* blood glucose level greater than 250 mg/dl are considered as diabetic animals and included in this study. The blood glucose levels, body weight, food, and water intake is measured on 2nd, 7th, 14th 21st, and 28th days [27 - 34].

3.12. Evaluation ofAnti-asthmatic Effect of Herbal Medicine

At the point when guinea pigs are presented to an aerosol containing histamine, it causes bronchoconstriction prompting asphyxia and death. Antihistamine medications anticipate or delay the hour of the beginning of attack by histamine aerosol. The death is continuing by dyspnea and spasm. The animal can be spared if the aerosol is speedily removed and stopped.The instrument comprises of a clear-cut box of Perspex isolated by perforated divided into two. There is little opening to spray aerosol. The spray is done utilizing a nebulizer which is associated with a sphygmomanometer and compressor. One side of the case that has a versatile segment is to expel aerosol [35]. Guinea pigs of indistinguishable weight are chosen for the investigations. One guinea pig that has received a saline solution is set in one chamber and marked as control. Another guinea pig got diphenhydramine (40 mg/kg body weight). The aerosol containing histamine is spread by nebulizer into the chamber and record the time till the animal (control) demonstrates dyspnea and seizure. The top is immediately opened to evacuate vaporized and the animal is permitted to recover. The animal treated with diphenhydramine (40 mg/kg) doesn't get spasms while saline-treated animal produces the seizure.

3.13. Evaluation of Locomotor Activity of Herbal Medicine

CNS acting drugs impact the locomotor action in animals. The CNS depressant property decreases the locomotor action while the stimulant property increases the locomotor action. The locomotor activity can be a index of alertness of mental action. The locomotor action (level of action) can be effectively assessed by an actophotometer, which works on photoelectric cells which are associated in circuit with a counter. A beam of light falling on the photocell is cut off by the animal, a count is automatically recorded. An actophotometer has either a circular field or square field in which the animal moves around. Both rats & mice may be employed for testing in this method [35, 36].

CONCLUSION

The main objectives of this book chapterto develop a standard protocol for the evaluation of plant-based drugs for the prevention and management of various clinical conditions. The fundamental basic scientific knowledge is essential to involve a new therapeutic regimen that should be safe and effective.To study the basic human physiology, which to understand the digestion, biotransformation, metabolism and excretion of the drugs are needed. Pharmacognostic and pharmacological evaluation cannot be done without sophisticated analytical equipment's like NMR and X-ray crystallography. In order to study the molecular mechanism, we need to study the genetic variation of the human body as well as different organ systems involved in drug metabolism. Without a pharmacokinetic study, it is difficult to assess the safety and efficacy profile of each of the herbal products. Recently most advanced tools are available to isolate the active ingredient and observed the structure and functional relationship and to study drug to drug interaction or drug to food interaction. Crossing the blood-brain barrier, and molecular study of various receptors involved in the therapeutic regimen. We have given the outline of certain experimental models to use some more advanced technique like high-throughput apparatus, an advanced version imagining of the various organ systems, and to decide the pathways involved in the disease as well as drugs acting on different organ systems. Readers are urged to indicate the references referenced for additional data and we trust that this material will be an important partner in our quest for a major comprehension in the most interesting region of pre-clinical information of pharmacology.

CONSENT FOR PUBLICATION

Not applicable.

CONFLICT OF INTEREST

None to be declared.

ACKNOWLEDGEMENTS

Declared none.

ABBREVIATIONS

CPK	Creatine phosphokinase
CPCSEA	Committee for the Purpose of Control and Supervision of Experiments in Animals
CNS	Central nervous system
HDL	High-density lipoprotein
HMG-CoA	β Hydroxy β-methylglutaryl-CoA
LDL	Low-density lipoprotein
LCAT	Lecithin cholesterol acyltransferase
mg/kg	Milligram per kilogram
P.O.	Per os (oral)
SGOT	Serum glutamic oxaloacetic transaminase
SGPT	Serum glutamic pyruvic transaminase
STZ	Streptozotocin
UI	Ulcer index

REFERENCES

[1]   Guide for the Care and Use of Laboratory Animals- Institute of Laboratory Animal Resources Commission on Life Sciences - National Research Council. Washington (DC). 8th ed., US: National

Academies Press 2011.

[2]   Hedrich H.J and Bullock G. The laboratory Mouse. London: Elsevier Academic Press 2004.

[3]   Jackson RK, Kieffer VA, Sauber JJ, King GL. A tethered-restraint system for blood collection from ferrets. Lab Anim Sci 1988; 38(5): 625-8.
        [PMID: 3193763]

[4]   Ormandy EH, Schuppli CA, Weary DM. Worldwide trends in the use of animals in research: the contribution of genetically-modified animal models. Altern Lab Anim 2009; 37(1): 63-8.
        [http://dx.doi.org/10.1177/026119290903700109] [PMID: 19292576]

[5]   Plummer JL, Cmielewski PL, Gourlay GK, Owen H, Cousins MJ. Assessment of antinociceptive drug effects in the presence of impaired motor performance. J Pharmacol Methods 1991; 26(1): 79-87.
        [http://dx.doi.org/10.1016/0160-5402(91)90057-C] [PMID: 1921412]

[6]   Kambur O, Männistö PT, Viljakka K, *et al.* Stress-induced analgesia and morphine responses are changed in catechol-O-methyltransferase-deficient male mice. Basic Clin Pharmacol Toxicol 2008; 103(4): 367-73.
        [http://dx.doi.org/10.1111/j.1742-7843.2008.00289.x] [PMID: 18834357]

[7]   Uthrapathy S, Shabi MM, Krishnamoorthy G, Ravindhran D, Rajamanickam VG, Dubey GP. Analgesic and anti-arthritic effect of *Corallocarpus epigaeus*. Acta Bioquim Clin Latinoam 2011; 45(4): 749-56.

[8]   Shabi MM, Uthrapathy S, Raj CD, *et al.* Analgesic and anti-arthritic effect of *Enicostemma littorale* Blume. Adv Biosci Biotechnol 2014; 5(10): 18-24.
        [http://dx.doi.org/10.4236/abb.2014.513116]

[9]   Winter CA, Risley EA, Nuss GW. Carrageenin-induced edema in hind paw of the rat as an assay for antiiflammatory drugs. Proc Soc Exp Biol Med 1962; 111: 544-7.
        [http://dx.doi.org/10.3181/00379727-111-27849] [PMID: 14001233]

[10]   Shabi MM, Dhevi R, Gayathri K, Subashini U, Rajamanickam GV, Dubey GP. C. Halicacabum (Linn): Investigations on anti-inflammatory and analgesic effect. Bulgarian J Veterinary Med 2009; 12(3): 171-7.

[11]   Vetriselvan S, Subasini U, Velmurugan C, Muthuramu T, Jothi S. Revathy. Anti-inflammatory activity of *Cucumis sativus* seed in Carrageenan and Xylene induced edema model using albino Wistar rats. Inter J Biopharm 2013; 4(1): 34-7.

[12]   Green K, Downs SJ. Ocular penetration of pilocarpine in rabbits. Arch Ophthalmol 1975; 93(11): 1165-8.
        [http://dx.doi.org/10.1001/archopht.1975.01010020871009] [PMID: 1191106]

[13]   Tripathi KD. Essential of medical pharmacology. New Delhi: Jaypee brothers 1999; p. 434.

[14]   Turner RA. Screening methods in pharmacology. New York: Academic Press 1965; p. 158.

[15]   Williamson EM, Okpoko DT, Evans FJ. Pharmacological methods in Phytotherapy Research. 155-67.

[16]   Liu X, Lee TL, Wong PT. Cyclooxygenase-1 inhibition shortens the duration of diazepam-induced loss of righting reflex in mice. Anesth Analg 2006; 102(1): 135-40.
        [http://dx.doi.org/10.1213/01.ane.0000189102.09347.2e] [PMID: 16368818]

[17]   Thatte U. Still in search of a herbal medicine. Indian J Pharmacol 2009; 41(1): 1-3.
        [http://dx.doi.org/10.4103/0253-7613.48876] [PMID: 20177572]

[18]   Rang HP, Dale MM, Ritter JM, Moore PK. Pharmacology. 5th ed. Churchill Livingston 2003; pp. 562-83.

[19]   Turner-Robert A. Screening Methods in Pharmacology. New York, London: Academic Press 1965.

[20]   Enna SJ. Short Protocols in Pharmacology and Drug Discovery. John Wiley and Sons Inc. 2007.

[21]   Kulkarni SK. Hand Book of Experimental Pharmacology, VallabhPrakashan, New Delhi. 1999; p. 125.

[22]   Subramaniam S, Ramachandran S, Uthrapathi S, Gnamanickam VR, Dubey GP. Anti-hyperlipidemic and antioxidant potential of different fractions of *Terminalia arjuna* Roxb. bark against PX- 407 induced hyperlipidemia. Indian J Exp Biol 2011; 49(4): 282-8.
[PMID: 21614892]

[23]   Saravanan S, Ramachandran S. Suja Rajapandian, Subasini U, Victor Rajamanickam G, Dubey GP. Anti-atherogenic activity of ethanolic fraction of *Terminalia arjuna* bark on hypercholesterolemic rabbits. Evid Based Complement Alternat Med 2011.
[http://dx.doi.org/10.1093/ecam/neq003]

[24]   Subasini U, Thenmozhi S, Venkateswaran V, Pavani P, Diwedi S, Rajamanickam VG. Phytochemical Analysis and Anti-hyperlipidemic Activity of *Nelumbo nucifera* in Male Wistar rats. InterJPharm Teach Pract 2014; 5(1): 935-40.

[25]   Subasini U, Thenmozhi S, Sathyamurthy D, Victor Rajamanickam G. Attenuation of fructose induced hyperlipidemia of *Enicostemma axillare*. Int J Pharm Phytopharmacol Res 2012; 1(5): 306-12.

[26]   Ahamad J, Amin S, Mir SR. Anti-hyperglycemic activity of charantin isolated from fruits of *Momordica charantia* Linn. Int Res J Pharm 2019; 10(1): 61-4.
[http://dx.doi.org/10.7897/2230-8407.100111]

[27]   Ahamad J, Hasan N, Amin S, Mir SR. Swertiamarin contributes to glucose homeostasis *via* inhibition of carbohydrate metabolizing enzymes. J Natural Rem 2016; 16(4): 125-30.

[28]   Ahamad J, Mir SR, Naquvi KJ. Hypoglycemic activity of aqueous extract of *Berberis aristata* stems bark in STZ-induced rats. InterJPharmPharmaSci 2012; 4(2): 473-4.

[29]   Naquvi KJ, Ali M, Ahamad J. Antidiabetic activity of aqueous extract of *Coriandrum sativum* L. fruits in streptozotocin induced rats. Int J Pharm Pharm Sci 2012; 4(1): 239-40.

[30]   Naquvi KJ, Ali M, Ahamad J. Antidiabetic and cholesterol lowering activities of the stem bark of *Ficus bengalensis* L. Natural Product An Indian J 2012; 8(8): 328-31.

[31]   Etuk EU. Animals models for studying diabetes mellitus. Agric Biol J N Am 2010; 1(2): 130-4.

[32]   Subramanian R, Asmawi MZ, Sadikun A. *In vitro* α-glucosidase and α-amylase enzyme inhibitory effects of *Andrographis paniculata* extract and andrographolide. Acta Biochim Pol 2008; 55(2): 391-8.
[http://dx.doi.org/10.18388/abp.2008_3087] [PMID: 18511986]

[33]   Subasini U, Shabi MM, Gayathri K, *et al*. Phytochemical evaluation with hypoglycaemic and antioxidant activity of *Tribulus terrestris* Linn. Inter J Biomed 2009; 29(2): 121-7.

[34]   Williamson EM, Okpoko DT, Evans FJ. Pharmacological methods in phytotherapy research. Third Avenue, New York, USA: John Wiley and sons, Inc. 1996; pp. 155-67.

[35]   Cao BJ, Rodgers RJ. Comparative effects of novel 5-HT1A receptor ligands, LY293284, LY315712 and LY297996, on plus-maze anxiety in mice. Psychopharmacology (Berl) 1998; 139(3): 185-94.
[http://dx.doi.org/10.1007/s002130050703] [PMID: 9784072]

[36]   Butterweck V. Mechanism of action of St John's wort in depression : what is known? CNS Drugs 2003; 17(8): 539-62.
[http://dx.doi.org/10.2165/00023210-200317080-00001] [PMID: 12775192]

[37]   Chen CR, Tan R, Qu WM, *et al*. Magnolol, a major bioactive constituent of the bark of *Magnolia officinalis*, exerts antiepileptic effects *via* the GABA/benzodiazepine receptor complex in mice. Br J Pharmacol 2011; 164(5): 1534-46.
[http://dx.doi.org/10.1111/j.1476-5381.2011.01456.x] [PMID: 21518336]

[38]   Harati E, Roodsari HRS, Seifi B, Kamalinejad M, Nikseresht S. The effect of oral *Matricaria chamomilla* extract and selenium on postpartum depression and plasma oxidant-anti-oxidant system in

mice. Tehran Univ Med J 2014; 71: 625-34.

[39] Machado DG, Cunha MP, Neis VB, *et al.* Antidepressant-like effects of fractions, essential oil, carnosol and betulinic acid isolated from *Rosmarinus officinalis* L. Food Chem 2013; 136(2): 999-1005.
[http://dx.doi.org/10.1016/j.foodchem.2012.09.028] [PMID: 23122155]

[40] Amrani S, Harnafi H, Bouanani NelH, *et al.* Hypolipidaemic activity of aqueous *Ocimum basilicum* extract in acute hyperlipidaemia induced by triton WR-1339 in rats and its antioxidant property. Phytother Res 2006; 20(12): 1040-5.
[http://dx.doi.org/10.1002/ptr.1961] [PMID: 17006976]

[41] Tuncer MA, Yaymaci B, Sati L, *et al.* Influence of *Tribulus terrestris* extract on lipid profile and endothelial structure in developing atherosclerotic lesions in the aorta of rabbits on a high-cholesterol diet. Acta Histochem 2009; 111(6): 488-500.
[http://dx.doi.org/10.1016/j.acthis.2008.06.004] [PMID: 19269683]

[42] Nader MA, el-Agamy DS, Suddek GM. Protective effects of propolis and thymoquinone on development of atherosclerosis in cholesterol-fed rabbits. Arch Pharm Res 2010; 33(4): 637-43.
[http://dx.doi.org/10.1007/s12272-010-0420-1] [PMID: 20422375]

CHAPTER 7

Product Development of Herbal Medicine

Ahmed Nawaz Khan[1,*], **Chandra Kala**[2] and **Javed Ahmad**[3]

[1] *School of Pharmacy, Graphic Era Hill University, Dehradun. Uttarakhand, 248002, India*

[2] *Faculty of Pharmacy, Maulana Azad University, Jodhpur, Rajasthan, 342802, India*

[3] *Department of Pharmaceutics, College of Pharmacy, Najran University, KSA*

Abstract: Treating diseases with medicinal plants is considered as the oldest therapeutic method that provides relief from illness to the whole humankind. In developing countries, a large group of the population have been found using phytotherapy for centuries, and still, they are following the same remedies. Preparation and compounding of one or more herbs containing phytochemicals lead to the production of finished herbal products, which are formulated from dried roots and extracts. Widespread use of these products requires quality and safety with good manufacturing practices and stringent evaluation criteria. From basic to advance, this chapter addresses the challenges and procedures ranging from harvesting, selection of plants, extraction, and formulation to the product approval by following the good agriculture, laboratory practice and good clinical practice and it would be a helpful medium for consideration during the product development period. As a whole, this chapter gives an overview to academicians, researchers, and industrial personnel for a better understanding of herbal products.

Keywords: Dosage Form, Good Manufacturing Practice, Herbal Products, Herbal Preparations, Phytochemicals, Phytoconstituents.

1. INTRODUCTION

Being healthy is the right of every human, and this right is a state of complete emotional and physical wellbeing that is necessary for living a happy life [1]. Additionally, when health gets disrupted by any weaknesses; nature serves with multiple interventions by its phytochemicals (in Greek phyto means plant). These phytochemicals are important for the growth, development, and protection of plants; and they also help in the cure of many human and veterinary diseases [2]. With good trust, these naturally occurring chemical moieties in plants are also responsible for the color, odor, and flavor; and are considered to be a major cont-

---

* **Corresponding author Ahmed Nawaz Khan:** School of Pharmacy, Graphic Era Hill University, Dehradun. Uttarakhand, India 248002; E-mail: ahmednawaz4u@gmail.com

Javed Ahmad and Javed Ahamad (Ed.)

ributor for protecting the health [3]. Phytochemical products are obtained from dried roots (herbal material) and extracts (herbal preparation) of the plant or herbs [4]. These plants contribute 11% of the drugs listed in 252 drugs of the World Health Organization's (WHO) essential medicines [5]. Surprisingly, there are about 121 bioactive phytochemicals commonly prescribed by the medical practitioners, which are among one-fourth of the drugs prescribed across the globe [6].

Treating diseases with medicinal plants is considered as the oldest therapy system that provides relief from illnesses to the humankind. In India, such systems are extensively followed through Ayurvedic, Unani, and Siddha system of medicine; and now Aamchi which also refers to as Tibetan Medicine System has also been included. Globally, these systems come under complementary medicines which are also referred to as integrating, naturopathy, or alternative medicine system [7]. Being therapeutically active, medicinal plants are used from Ayurveda to Chinese traditional medicines, Unani to Aamchi and Amazonian to African medicines, *etc.*, which integrate phytotherapy in these systems irrespective of their versatile theoretical and cultural values [8]. Such alternatives may provide an authentic and efficacious therapeutic treatment in case of many incurable diseases; and can help practitioners to accept a new and interesting line of treatment. Along with the right to choose treatment methods or therapies; in general, people are free to select bioactive phytochemicals products or phytomedicines on a self-selection basis. Day by day, demand for herbal products is increasing due to growing consumers' interest in alternative or natural therapies [9]. More than three fourth of the Indian population prefer phytochemical products for treatment, [10] moreover, up to 90% of Africans depend on traditional medicines and surprisingly traditional medicines in China account for 40% of the health delivery system [11]. However, with a new framework of evidence-based medicines; the development of these traditional products becomes a challenge for pharmaceutical industries. Under the correct scientific and ethical standards for research and development, there are big challenges like lack of scientific validation and standardization, lack of quality and regulatory aspects, limited evidence-based studies on efficacy and safety, and lack of pharmacokinetic studies of bioactive compounds Thus scientific validity of herbal products is still often questioned. Besides these challenges and to understand the herbal product development, this chapter highlights current issues and gives insights into harvesting and regulatory procedures, including clinical and nonclinical aspects, for the development of bioactive herbal products.

1.1. Scope of Herbal Medicinal Products

Consumption of phytochemical products declined when synthetic medicines evolved; however, for the past few decades, phytotherapy is again booming in all industrialized countries. Interestingly in developing countries, a large group of the population has been found to use phytotherapy for centuries, and still, they are following the same remedies. It has been observed that when synthetic medicines proved ineffective in chronic diseases like cancer or new infectious diseases, the demand for these herbal products increased [12]. Furthermore, continuing research on ethnobotanics is leading to the discovery of new phytochemicals present in nature for the treatment of various major pathologies and are opening new ways for drug development [13]. Due to affordability, fewer side effects, and easy accessibility even without prescription make these phytochemical products highly acceptable by the consumer.

2.   CHALLENGES   IN   HERBAL   MEDICINAL   PRODUCT DEVELOPMENT

Phytochemical products have reached extensive acceptability across the globe as therapeutic and nutritional products. However, quantitative and qualitative analysis of the phytochemical composition of bioactive compounds or markers is a major challenge. Science admits that consuming food rich in these chemical compounds has health benefits however, pieces of evidence exist to prove the specific recommendation for these phytochemical intakes. Even there are some known health effects of phytochemicals that researchers have not recognized yet. Moreover, it is known that 'Herbal product is free of side effects', but this is not completely true [14]; as many extensive scientific studies reject this myth. Clinical data reveals the real picture like cardiovascular ailments with the use of ephedra, hepatotoxicity by kava-kava consumption, and water retention by licorice [15, 16]. Many other studies have reported numbers of side effects and adverse reactions in consumers for a wide range of mechanisms [9]. In a WHO database, 4 million reports from 100 countries across the globe are indicated out of which 21,000 discussed the adverse effects of natural products [17]. Another study from American Poison Centres revealed that a user consuming supplements, herbal and homeopathy products fell into a category which was linked to hospital admission [18, 19]. These Adverse Drug Reactions (ADR) negatively affect the promotion of herbal products, and the most common reason of these adverse drug reactions is attributed to the presence of adulterants, undeclared substances, synthetic chemicals, or some other active ingredients which are common during product development or trading of raw medicinal plants [6]. The adulteration sometimes is unintended and may be due to the case of substitution between various Indian traditional systems of medicine. For instance, 'Parpatta' in Ayurveda sounds similar to 'Parpadagam' in the Siddha system of medicine, both of which refer to a different drug, carry the chances of adulteration or substitution with each other [6]. These evidence prepare regulatory agencies of many countries to bring out alerts on monitoring the quality of herbal product strictly. Therefore involvement of patients for the course of pharmacovigilance reporting is another big challenge like there are under-reporting adverse reactions for herbal derivatives or synthesized drugs [9]. Two studies in the United Kingdom and Italy showed that 69% and 61.7% of users respectively failed to inform serious or minor adverse events from herbal products to their medical consultant. Therefore, during the clinical risk assessment of herbal-product, the first step is the correct identification and assessment of risk through the examination of the patient and available scientific evidence. The presence of risk factors for the herbal products to the consumers is expected to be evaluated - while this may be difficult being imperative since these factors can determine a reaction's severity and incidence. For this reason, India being one of the largest consumers of herbal products, the pharmacovigilance is on demand to cover side effects and adverse reactions for the safety concerns of patients and users. Thus it is important for health professionals to follow a thorough process by keeping in mind the scientific, pharmacological, and toxicological knowledge.

Another concern before product development is herbal material, which is likely to get contaminated by various fungi while harvesting, handling, storage, production, and distribution. Less monitored and unchecked harvesting of plant species results in depletion and affects the quality of phytochemicals such as crude medicinal plants and their preparations are reported to contain pesticide residues as contaminants. A report from Traditional Chinese Medicines (TCM) revealed the presence of pesticides like Organo Chlorine Pesticides (OCPs) [21]. The pesticide content in the herbal materials affects the progress and global acceptance of herbal medicines. To deal with the above problem, the WHO established a suitable method of detection of pesticides in herbal materials and their maximum residue limits (MRL). Various countries provide the methods for detection and residual limits for OCPs through their pharmacopeia. It has also been reported in studies conducted in 2003 that approximately 20% of herbal drugs imported to the United States of America (USA) by India and Pakistan contained a high amount of heavy metals such as arsenic, lead, and mercury [22]. Furthermore, in 2008, a study showed 21.7% of the USA manufactured ayurvedic medicines, and 19.5% of products from India sold on the internet, to be carrying heavy elements like arsenic, lead, and mercury [23]. Therefore, herbal products must be monitored properly. Fig. (1) shows the evaluation stages for the quality of the herbal drug.

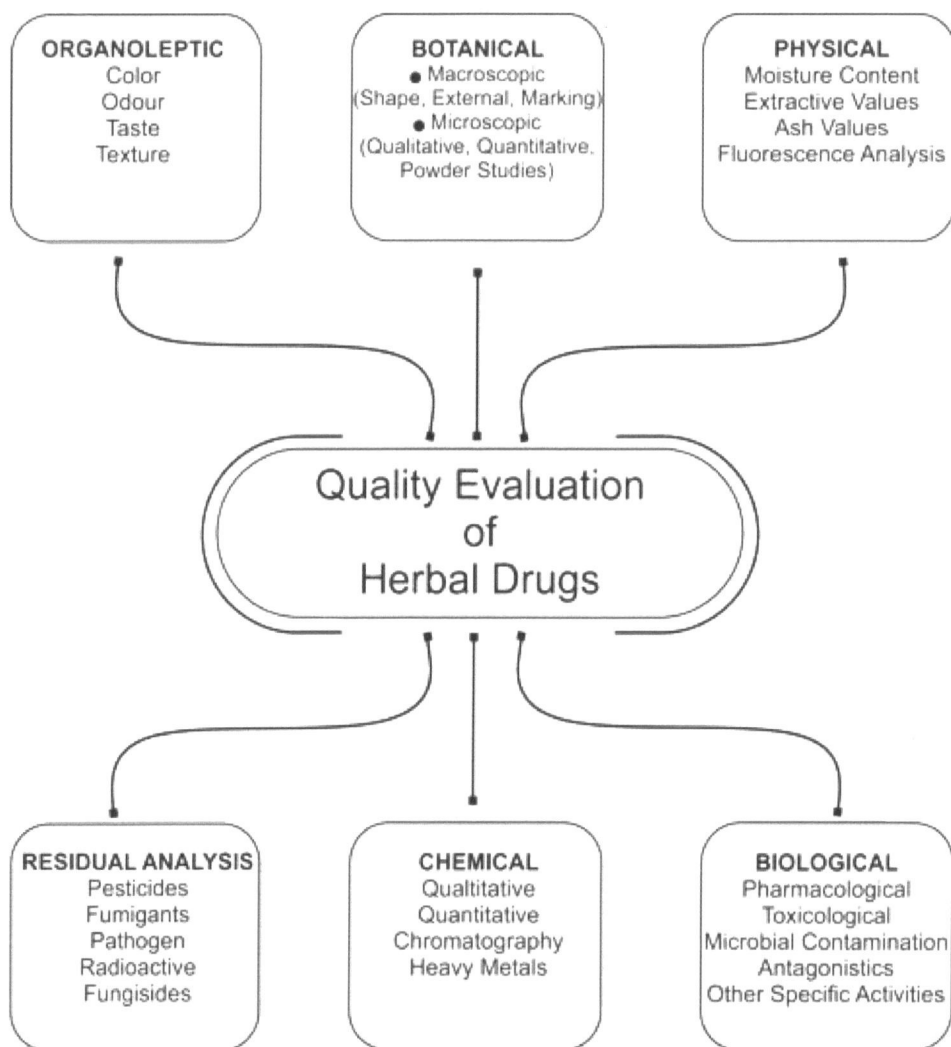

Fig. (1). Quality evaluation of herbal drugs.

Another important challenge is the processing of a herbal material that is derived from the same plant species by different methods, which plays an important role during product development. Some differences in quality and therapeutic properties may also be seen. For instance, unprocessed raw licorice is used as expectorant and antitussive; but on stirring and frying with honey, it changes into a tonic, which helps in replenishing the body strength. One more big challenge associated with these products is knowing all ingredients of the extract, which can differ due to cultivation techniques, collection processes, extraction methods, production compliance, and incorrect identification of herbs, *etc.* [24]. For addressing the complexity and intrinsic variability of the ingredients present in herbal extracts, a recent article suggest that the problem of suspected adulteration and pollution can be resolved by applying the rigid standards of Good Manufacturing Practice (GMP) and Good Agricultural and Collection Practices (GACP) to the field of herbal remedies and supplements [25]. Fig. (**2**) depicts the complete development line from plant to product. Along with GMP and GACP, Good Laboratory Practice (GLP), and Good Clinical Practice (GCP) guidelines; processing concerns demand the development of new methods that certify the quality, purity, and safety of the herbal drug and its product.

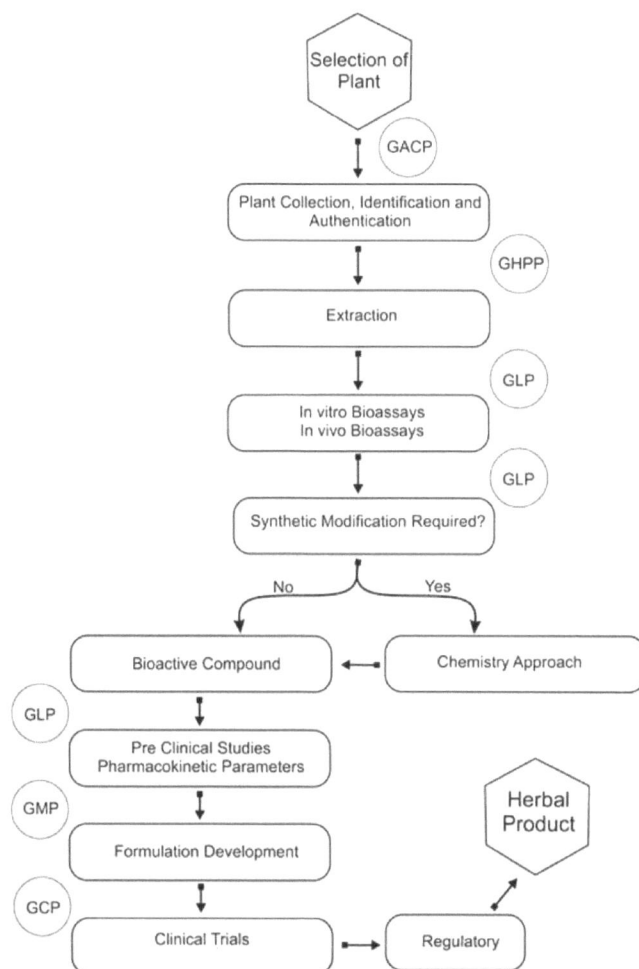

Fig. (2). Development line from plant to product following GACP (Good Agriculture and Collection Practice), GHPP (Good Herbal Processing Practice), GLP (Good Laboratory Practice), GMP (Good Manufacturing Practice), and GCP (Good Clinical Practice).

3. DOSAGE FORMS OF HERBAL MEDICINAL PRODUCTS

Phytochemicals are derived from herbs. These herbs come from entire plant or fragmented parts of plant, and sometimes powder form of a plant part like leaf, fruit, seed, stem, and bark, *etc.* Once processed by steaming and roasting, they are converted in the form of fresh juices, gums, fixed oils, essential oils, and resins; or sometimes kept unprocessed in the form of dry powder of herbs; such material is considered as herbal material. And when extraction, fractionation, purification, and other biological methods are applied to them to make an extract, tincture, and fatty oils, they are referred to as herbal preparations [26]. Preparation and compounding of one or more herbs turn them into finished herbal products. With the advancement in science, compounds or phytoconstituents can be easily isolated from plants and tested against diseases. These compounds can be synthetically prepared and consumed for the curing of disease. But these chemically defined active chemicals in the form of synthetic chemicals or single isolated compound from plant material cannot be considered as "herbal" [4].

Herbal drugs or phytochemical products in the market are mainly categorized into four classes [6, 25]:

Indigenous Herbal Medicine: These are dosage forms of historical use with well-known composition for the various treatments.

Herbal Medicine: These have been traditionally used in Ayurveda, Unani, and Siddha system of medicine for a long time. For such products, efficacy is not generally required.

Modified Herbal Medicine: These are prepared by modifications in indigenous herbal medicine or herbal medicine in dosage form; thereby changing the route of administration, ingredient composition, preparation method, and indications. Such products must meet the safety and efficacy criteria as drafted by the national regulatory authorities of the country of origin. Moreover, after modification(s), clinical data and preclinical data may or may not be prerequisites for this class.

Imported Product with an Herbal Base: These are pre-registered and marketed products from countries of origin with safety and efficacy data which is imported and submitted to the importing country.

Dosage forms of phytochemical products are broadly categorized into solid, liquid, and semisolid; with or without excipients [4] and they are as follows:

3.1. Solid Dosage Form

Solid dosage forms are prepared by bioactive phytochemical material or a combination of multiple phytochemicals in the form of powder or granules, *etc.* They contain permissible suitable excipients such as binding agent, disintegrator, glidant, anti-adherent, coating agent, sweetener, lubricant, and flavouring agent, *etc.* Here are some examples:

Herbal Tea Bag is used as an infusion which may contain an herb or a mixture of different herbs. For making this product; a herbal material like dried roots, leaves, or flowers is kept inside a paper or cloth bag. This bag material must be free of gluten, bleach, and dioxin. For sealing the bag, thread stitching is required but no metallic pins are used due to the possibility of releasing harmful cations into the infusion.

Plant Powder is one of the most common solid dosage forms. This is available in fine size or coarse particles form. No nano size powder comes under this category. During preparation dried herbal material is grinded and pulverised; which further convert into a suitable particle size. And finally powder can be used as such or get packed in capsules or sachets.

Dry Extract Powders are obtained by evaporating the solvent during extraction process. Most adoptable ways are spray drying or freeze-drying techniques. These methods are used on a fluid extract with or without using adsorbent like methylcellulose. Dry extract powder has a powdery consistency; and contains stabilizers and preservatives to make stable dosage form. Excipients also introduced for improving the taste and make the packaging easy. This type is used as such or compressed into tablets or filled in capsules.

Granules are the fluid extract or dried liquid extract prepared by agglomerations of small particles into spherical particles. First, a fluid extract is blended with binders, diluents, or some excipients; then on wetting with appropriate binding solvent it turns to agglomeration. Finally it is dried and separated into desired sizes. These granules can be used as such or compressed into tablets or filled in capsules shells.

Pills are a spherical solid form of dry extract powders which are much greater than granules size. Extract powder is blended with suitable dried excipients or liquid excipients for binding and providing plasticity to make proper mass form.

Capsules encompass the phytochemical constituents in the hard or soft gelatin capsule shells. Generally non-hygroscopic solid dried plant powder or homogenous dry extract and sometimes granules with suitable excipients are directly filled in hard gelatin capsules. While hygroscopic materials of liquid extract must be used in liquid form and encapsulated in a soft gelatin capsule shell.

Tablets are the compressed form of plants' powder or granules combined with excipients like binders and diluents. This dosage form can be prepared in different shapes and sizes by using compression; and finally may get coated or uncoated as required.

Lozenges or troches are prepared by cooking herbal extract with excipients like sucrose or sorbitol in water. On cooling; flavoring agents are added and uniformly mixed. Then molten mass is filled into molds. Packing must be thick to avoid moisture absorption so that sugar base remains safe from crystallization.

3.2. Liquid Dosage Form

Liquid dosage form is prepared by adding herbal material in an aqueous or non-aqueous solvent; or by making one or two-phase of oil and water system. This form may contain appropriate excipients such as antioxidants, preservatives, buffering agents, wetting agents, solubilizing agents, flavoring agents, sweetener, and coloring agents which are approved by the regulatory body. Here are some examples:

A *fluid extract* is prepared by the percolation method used on herbal material(s) with aqueous-alcohol menstruum in such a way that 1 ml of fluid extract contains 1 g of herbal extract. This must be thoroughly moistened and packed into a percolator with more menstruum. Keeping for 24 hours on maceration and percolated at a moderate rate, then some additional menstruum is added to make soft extract at a temperature of not more than 60°C. Preserve the first 700-800 ml of the percolate as reserved and used when the residue of additional percolate is concentrated. Finally, make this filtered if required.

A *decoction* is prepared by boiling herbal material with water or aqueous ethanol and sometime glycerol. Commonly this is a water-based preparation. The automatic decocting machine is used which works on a specific temperature for specific duration. Decoction is filled in airtight sealed plastic pouches as a single dose unit. For hard and woody plant parts like seeds, roots, stems, and rhizome; decoction is preferred. First, the plant material is dried and grinded into the powdered form. In case of using fresh plant material, it has to be cut down into small portions or used in crush form. Dried herbs are used equivalent to 1 teaspoon and fresh herb as 1 tablespoon per 250 ml of water. It is recommended to start the process with cold water as it facilitates the extraction of plant constituents before the coagulation of other plant constituents such as proteins that can block the extraction of constituents. The mixture is then boiled over medium flame for 20 minutes or until the volume of water is reduced by half.

An *Infusion* is prepared by macerating the herbal material in water for a short time. This can also be prepared in vinegar or edible oil. When soft and woody herbs are used for preparation, it is preferred to prepare infusion and decoction separately before mixing to facilitate the most effective extraction. And if the herb is containing a high percentage of volatile oils, it is preferred to make a fine powder of the herb and use the infusion method.

A *tincture* is prepared in the alcoholic or hydro-alcoholic medium (like ethanol and water) in a ratio of 1 part herbal material and 5-10 parts of solvent.

Syrups are prepared by using a solution of honey, sucrose, or some other appropriate sweetening agent. For making syrups; herbal extract is dissolved, mixed, suspended, or emulsified and heated in a minimum amount of 45% m/m of sweetening agent. Further water is added to make the syrup of desired weight; and suitable preservative is also added to prevent the bacterial growth.

Emulsions are prepared by at least two immiscible liquid such as oil-in-water preparation with the use of emulsifying agent(s) which make the emulsion stabilized and homogenized. One liquid is uniformly dispersed in another immiscible liquid in the form of small droplets and an interface appears between oily and aqueous phase. Emulsification of this preparation is done through agitators, homogenizers, colloid mills, and ultrasonic devices. For instance, castor oil in water preparation emulsified with gum acacia.

Aromatic waters are prepared by water preparations which are saturated with essential oils or other aromatic or volatile substances. Commonly 1 part of essential oil is mixed with 999 parts of fresh distilled water along with 10 parts of talcum powder; and stands the preparation for 12 hours or more. Aromatic water always must be made in small quantities for immediate use because aromatic water may deteriorate over time due to decomposition, mold growth, or volatilization. Thus, this preparation must be stored in an airtight container away from light and heat.

3.3. Semi-Solid Dosage Forms

Ointments and Creams are the semisolid preparation for topical use. Herbal powder or extract are taken with appropriate base and emulsifier or thickening agents. Then all are heated, mixed, and stirred well to achieve a viscosity of semisolid form. If preparation is required to keep for longer time then adding a preservative is necessary. Otherwise, the preservative may or may not be used.

Plaster and patches comprise of herbal preparation are in the form of the dry or soft extract on a sheet of plastic elastomer or a fibre piece that give support and adherence towards the skin and providing back support.

Medicated oils are prepared using fixed oils which are macerated or boiled with herbal extract or juice. Powder or extract in water or milk is mixed with oil and macerated or boiled steadily to remove moisture or water. For decanting or straining the oil; muslin cloth is used and thereafter oil is cooled.

4. RECOMMENDATIONS IN HERBAL MEDICINAL PRODUCT DEVELOPMENT

Herbal drug preparations are comprised of variety of products such as powdered herbal drugs, tinctures, extracts, essential oils, expressed juices and process exudates; and these all are obtained through various treatments like extraction, distillation, expression, fractionation, purification, concentration and fermentation of the herbal drugs [27]. Efficient regulation of herbal drugs demands appropriate research data, control mechanisms, expertise from the manufacturers, which can only be collected during the product development phase. For example, during the standardization of an active phytochemical or combination of phytochemicals; processes must ensures the product to be safe and more effective for consumers [28]. There are no harmonized guidelines on herbal product development. However, the WHO has released the chain of documents and technical procedures as the extensive guidelines for herbal products such as 'Quality Control Methods for Medicinal Plant Materials', 'Guidelines on good agricultural and collection practices' (GACP) for medicinal plants in 2003 and 'WHO guidelines for assessing the quality of herbal medicines with reference to contaminants and residues' in 2007. These guidelines are for the purpose to assure safety, quality and efficacy of herbal medicinal plants and materials. Thus for better quality and effectiveness; manufacturers must follow these WHO guidelines along with Good Herbal Processing Practice (GHPP) and Good Manufacturing Practice (GMP) for Herbals by WHO. According to WHO, herbal medicines include herbs, herbal materials, herbal preparations, and finished herbal products of parts of the plant or their combination containing the active ingredient.

Furthermore, as per European Medicine Agency (EMEA), these herbal drug include whole plant, cut plant and fragmented plant or its part, unprocessed algae, fungi, lichen (in the dried or fresh state), and unprocessed exudates. Like WHO, EMEA has also introduced several guidelines on the assessment of quality, safety, efficacy, and non-clinical aspects of herbal medicines [29]. The Committee on Herbal Medicinal Products (HMPC) which is under EMEA has developed a simplified registration process that allows the registration of herbal medicinal products without certifications on safety and efficacy tests and trials. And this possible only if the evidences support that the product has been used for its medicinal value for at least 30 years with at least 15 years of period in the community (Article 16c (1) (c) of Directive 2001/83/EC).

In USA, most of the herbal products are considered as dietary supplements and are regulated under the Dietary Supplement Health and Education Act of 1994. They consider them as Botanical Drug Product, which is defined as a product prepared from raw botanical materials derived from one or more plants, algae, or macroscopic fungi. Some processes which are used for their preparation include pulverization, decoction, expression, aqueous and ethanolic extraction, or any other similar process, for its use as a medicine as per Section 201(g)(1)(B), Federal Food, Drug, and Cosmetic Act. In the USA, the botanical drug product may be marketed as an approved New Drug Application (NDA) or Over the Counter (OTC) drug monograph (21 CFR parts 331–358). Unlike synthetic medications, herbal supplements are not usually regulated stringently; and even are not go through the same scientific procedures as synthetic medication. Moreover, manufacturers are not required for placing their products in the markets with the approval of the Food and Drug Administration; however, they have to follow GMP guidelines. During labeling of primary packaging, manufacturers can not mention medical claims; however, however they can print nutritional value or health supporting research with a disclaimer that this product has not been evaluated by United States Food and Drug Administration (USFDA).

In India, herbal medicinal products are regulated in accordance with the Department of Ayurveda, Yoga & Naturopathy, Unani, Siddha, and Homoeopathy (AYUSH). They follow Schedule T of Drugs & Cosmetics Act, 1940; that deals with the rules for production and marketing of Ayurveda, Siddha, and Unani (ASU) drugs and even GMP of ASU drugs [31]. In the whole development phase of phytochemicals from cultivation to finished product, products undergo several challenges and filters. Qualifying all tests and procedures; a product results in a safe and effective product for consumption.

Good manufacturing practice is the principal system to measure the manufacturing process of these products. Therefore, taking WHO guidelines as a reference, national health authorities of all countries should establish their own current GMP requirement depending upon their circumstances [32]. For many years WHO has been engaged in the development of series of technical guidelines and upgrading of the existing guidelines associated with the quality assurance and these techniques assist in the identification of phytochemical constituents. Chemical makers used are classified into active markers and analytical markers. Active markers are those molecules or groups of molecules which are responsible for the therapeutic effects of the herbal medicinal product; while analytical markers are molecules or groups of molecules which are principally aid for analytical purposes.

1. *Extraction:* For extraction a suitable method must be adopted among decoction, infusion, maceration, percolation, supercritical fluid extraction, *etc.*
2. *Specification:* Products are of varying characteristics ranging from simple; comminuted plant material to extracts, resins, tinctures, and oils. Thus product specifications are directly linked to many parameters like definition (solvent used for extraction and drug extract ratio), quality, method of preparation, phytoconstituents with known therapeutic activity and stability profile. Other considerations which are important during preclinical and clinical trials are analytical markers, identification, assay, limit tests, and safety with efficacy of product batches. Hence, utilizing recent scientific data, a detailed specification must be undertaken for each phytochemical product.

Quality Control: Quality of herbal drugs directly influences their safety and efficacy. Therefore to warrant the herbal medicinal product consistency, the concept of 'Phytoequivalence' was introduced by Germany, where the chemical profile of the herbal medicinal drug in question is compared with the reference product whose chemical profile is clinically proven [34]. Contrarily, conventional quality control techniques are considered inadequate in determining the safety and efficacy of the herbal medicinal product and their identification or authentication. This insufficiency of conventional quality control techniques is attributed to the variation and complexities of the herbal medicinal products.

Below are some general attributes and recommended test which are required for the development of all phytochemical products:

a. *Definition:* It includes an explanation of the botanical source and product preparation type (*e.g.* liquid or dried extract). Herbs used must be mentioned accurately with their ratios.
b. *Characteristics:* A qualitative characterization of the organoleptic properties of the herbs is a prerequisite before formulation development starts.
c. *Identification:* A herbal preparation should have a specific identification test and ideally should be differential with respect to certain substitutes/adulterants. Identification using a single technique is not sufficient, and it is preferable to use a combination of chromatographic techniques such as HPLC and TLC or

TLC-densitometry or other techniques combination such as HPLC/MS, or GC/MS or HPLC/UV-diode array, whichever is more accountable as per requirement.

d. Recommended Tests

1. *Water content:* Hygroscopic herbal preparation must undergo this test. The result values for the effects of moisture absorption and hydration must satisfy the acceptance criteria. On one side, during product development, the effect of absorbed moisture versus water of hydration must be well characterized, like loss on drying test is considered sufficient for the determination of water content. However, in some instances, such as preparation containing essential oil; a water-specific detection procedure is required, like Karl Fischer titration.

2. *Impurities:* They are many inorganic impurities or toxic (heavy) metals present in the product; and determining these impurities must be considered relevant for product quality. Based on the understanding of plant species (wild or cultivated) and the manufacturing process, test procedure and acceptance criteria need to be accurate and precise for the detection of inorganic impurities during development.

3. *Microbial limits:* Total count of aerobic microorganisms, yeasts and mold, and the absence of specific harmful bacteria may be specified when required. Pharmacopoeial procedures or other validated procedures should be followed for microbial counts.

4. *Assay:* Assay of the content of product containing constituents of established therapeutic activities is required with the comprehensive analytical procedure. Wherever possible, the content of the herbal substance/s in the product should be determined using a specific and stability-indicating procedure. In case of a non-specific assay is justified, the overall specificity may be achieved by other supporting analytical procedures. For instance, during the assay of anthraquinone glycoside, an UltraViolet/Visible spectrophotometric procedure is followed with a suitable test for identification, *e.g.* chromatography which can be used in combination.

5. *Uniformity of mass:* For single-dose (dried powder) and multiple-dose (syrup) products uniformity test is to be followed. Acceptance criteria should be set for the volume of fill, and/or fill uniformity and variation of weight. If appropriate, tests may be carried out as in-process control. Nonetheless, the acceptance criteria should be comprehended in the specification or the formulation monograph.

6. *pH:* Acidity or basicity of the product must be known and justified.

7. *Microbial limits:* For the purpose of quality assurance of underdevelopment product, microbial testing is an attribute of Good

Manufacturing Practice. In order to avoid a significant risk of microbial contamination, total count of aerobic bacteria, the total count of yeasts and molds, and the absence of objectionable micro-organisms like *Staphylococcus aureus*, *Escherichia coli*, *Salmonella*, and *Pseudomonas* must be checked and determined by pharmacopoeial or other validated procedures.

8. *Antimicrobial preservative content:* For oral liquid dosage form, antimicrobial preservatives are prerequisites. Adding criteria should be based on the levels necessary to sustain microbiological product quality during the shelf-life. The minimum added concentration of antimicrobial preservatives should be tested and justified to be effective in controlling microorganisms.

9. *Antioxidant preservative content:* It is preferable to perform releasing test for antioxidant content. In some situations, it is confirmed by stability and method development testing. Shelf-life testing may be considered as inessential; and in-process testing may be required rather than release testing.

10. *Dissolution:* For soluble and sparingly soluble phytoconstituents of the product, a dissolution test should be followed and must lie under the acceptance criteria of the dosage form. If possible, it is recommended to follow the pharmacopeia or otherwise justified for testing apparatus, media, and conditions for the test. The dissolution procedure should be validated in both pharmacopoeial and non-pharmacopoeial procedures with respect to apparatus and conditions.

11. *Particle size distribution:* A procedure for the determination of particle size distribution must be appropriate for oral suspensions; and should come under the acceptance criteria specified in monograph of the formulation mentioned in pharmacopeia. Developmental data should be considered when determining the need for either a dissolution procedure or a particle size distribution procedure for these formulations. For example, it is appropriate to include quantitative analysis for the determination of particle size distribution in oral dosage form like suspensions.

12. *Redispersibility:* Liquid dosage form like suspension must have redispersibility. When product content settles down on storage, shaking is the appropriate way for redispersibility. The time required to attain re-suspension during manual or mechanical shaking must be clearly stated.

13. *Pharmacokinetic and pharmacodynamic study*: Pharmacological action of phytochemical(s) for therapeutic effect along with herb-food, herb-herb and drug-herb interaction must be studied. Thus pharmacodynamic (PD) study is conducted which is a non-clinical process and helps in ensuring safety for the consumers and elucidating the mechanism of action [35].

However, the physiological effect and mechanism of action of traditional medicine are still ambivalent and controversial [36]. Therefore along with pharmacodynamic study for a single herb or combination of herbs; pharmacokinetic (PK) study is also investigated for absorption, distribution, metabolism, and excretion of active phytochemical(s). Such a PK-PD model is suggested by many researchers [37] and therefore it must be followed appropriately. But due to the complexity of the multiple phytochemicals in the product, such study is a challenging task.

14. *Stability study*: Checking stability during the development phase is a prerequisite before filing product dossier due to the phytochemical complexity and variability in herbal composition. Therefore, to check the shelf life and impact of temperature, humidity; stability is recommended under the national and international guidelines [38]. Instability may also occur due to physical instability, chemical instability, environmental condition, decomposition, or storage. Thus many research studies suggest several methods to deal with instability issue; like nanoparticle coating or liposomes for protecting from enzymatic attack. This can happen by using polymeric plant-derived excipients (plant polysaccharides), chelating agents (polyvinylpyrrolidone) for stabilization of aqueous plant extract and liquid preparation coated with water-soluble cellulose derivative, *etc.* [39]. Stability will help the manufacturer to provide safer and effective long-term stable products that will help in gaining their confidence in the phytochemicals.

15. *Pre-clinical study*: All phytoconstituents used in the formulation must be safe and non-toxic. And after formulation, the preclinical study of the product is performed as per WHO guidelines [26]. Under the acute toxicity study male and female rodents and non-rodents are selected, and a sufficient number of doses level are tested in one or more doses for up to 24 hours. While in long term toxicity, an equal number of male and female rodent and non-rodent species are selected. During the administration period for long term toxicity; the study can be started from 2 weeks for a single dose, up to 12 months for long term repeated administration of the phytochemical preparation.

16. *Clinical Trials for evaluating safety and efficacy*: There is a lack of well-controlled double-blind clinical toxicological studies to establish the safety and efficacy of the herbal medicinal drugs, thus randomized clinical trials can be used as a safety tool during the development of bioactive phytochemical products. As for the synthetic chemicals, clinical studies require clinical trials in four different phases; phytochemical products are also recommended to undergo the clinical trials. WHO and many countries have their own clinical guidelines [35], however, in India there are no such

official guidelines [40]. So it would be better to follow the WHO guidelines. As per WHO, clinical trials have two purposes, one is to validate the safety and efficacy of the phytochemical product and the second is to develop or examine new indications of product, change of dosage form, or route of administration [35]. Thus clinical trials are conducted in four phases under the monitoring committee known as Ethics Review Board who follow the World Medical Association's Declaration of Helsinki. Following the clinical trials processes; quality assurance of botanical and herbal preparation is required which demands certification based on several parameters such as identification, water content, chemical assay of active ingredients, inorganic impurities (toxic metals), microbial limits, mycotoxins, pesticides, dissolution test, unit dosage uniformity, *etc.* It must be noted that chemistry, manufacturing, and control (CMC) documents for botanical and herbal medicines are very different from those which are provided for synthetic or highly purified drugs.

CONCLUSION AND FUTURE DIRECTIONS

With the increase in demand and use of herbal medicines, the global market is constantly expanding, and the safety and quality of herbal material and its finished product remain a major concern for the health authorities, pharmaceutical industries, and the consumers. It is observed that drug/medicine regulatory systems of several countries still lack the strict guidelines on evaluating and monitoring safety, efficacy, and quality control of traditional medicine/complementary and alternative medicine (TM/CAM).

Irrespective of health benefits and curing effect of phytochemical, less evidence suggest whether bioactivity is a result of single phytochemical or the interaction of various phytochemicals. Quality control requirements and methods for finished herbal products or phytochemical combination products are too complex as compared to the chemical/synthetic drugs. This complexity of phytochemicals is due to plant family, their potential interactions, and the possible variations in chemical levels found in any given product make this currently impossible to draft the specific phytochemical guidelines.

At present, it is well accepted that the good quality of the herbal medicines determines their safety and efficacy. Therefore, GMP is a principle step in warranting the safety and efficacy of herbal medicines. For satisfying the GMP requirements, manufacturers need big investments, and this may impose difficulty for small manufacturers, especially in developing countries. Such a situation may also lead to an increase in production costs which ultimately leads to an increase in the final product cost; and hence affordability of the products to consumers remains a challenge. Therefore, health authorities need to take relevant steps to motivate and ensure that the manufacturers are ready and capable of improving their GMP.

During product development, manufacturers must fulfil GMP for ensuring the consistent processing of the product and meeting quality standards. The purpose of good compliance is to make sure that the right ingredients in appropriate amounts are included; and harmful ingredients and contamination sources are kept out of the product. Moreover, thousands of bioactive phytochemicals have been extracted and tested through research; however, many are still to be discovered. Therefore for the development of new products in the market, pharmacodynamic result, stability study result, preclinical, and clinical study data along with the quality specification of the product must be analysed by globally harmonised guidelines to get the worldwide market approval of the product.

ABBREVIATIONS

ASU   Ayurveda, Siddha and Unani

AYUSH Ayurveda, Yoga & Naturopathy, Unani, Siddha and Homoeopathy

CAM   Complementary and Alternative Medicine

CMC   Chemistry, Manufacturing and Control

EMEA   European Medicine Agency

GACP   Good Agricultural and Collection Practices

GC   Gas Chromatography

GHPP   Good Herbal Processing Practice

GMP   Good Manufacturing Practice

HMPC   Committee on Herbal Medicinal Products

HPLC   High Performance Liquid Chromatography

MRL   Maximum Residue Limits

NDA   New Drug Application

OCPs   Organo Chlorine Pesticides

PD   Pharmacodynamics

PK   Pharmacokinetic

TCM   Traditional Chinese Medicines

TM   Traditional Medicine

TLC   Thin Layer Chromatography

USA   United States of America

USFDA United States Food and Drug Administration

UV   Ultra Violet

control of herbal medicines. And this is just to improve and promote the quality of herbal medicine and reducing the proportion of adverse effects associated with the poor quality of herbal medicines.

Monitoring of the manufacturing process is essential as it is one of the major steps where quality control is needed for assuring the quality of herbal medicines [32]. To make a product safer and effective; here are some general guidelines for the development of bioactive phytochemicals product [33]:

1. Selection of targeted disease and disorder.
2. Appropriate plant(s) selection whose pharmacological activity has been reported for targeted disease or disorder.
3. *Herb screening:* Either organically or biologically grown herbs; both are prone to contamination from the soil [8]. Conditions of harvesting, production, marketing, distribution of plant species, and factors such as soil conditions, climate, and moisture, *etc.* influence the chemical profile of the plant species. And therefore any possible contamination which may consider as potential risk must be dealt with more attention. It must be noted that the content of secondary metabolites of plants also get affected by several factors like time of cultivation, storage, drying, extraction, processing, and even packaging. Owing to all these effects, a detailed understanding of biological, chemical, genetic, and agronomic aspects of plant systems is primarily required. Thus it is important to maintain the chemical stability of the herbal material at all stages of the manufacturing process that verify the medicinal efficacy and consumer safety.
4. *Characterisation:* Detailed characterization of herbal substance/preparation or an herbal medicinal product; evaluation of botanical and phytochemical properties of the plant is required. For characterization acceptance criterion and details of specific herb; concerned values must be followed like in WHO guidelines or Ayurvedic Pharmacopoeia of India or Unani Pharmacopoeia of India that must be consulted for:

   ○ *Macroscopical/microscopical characterisation*
   ○ *Phytochemical characterisation*
   ○ *Impurities*
   ○ *Biological variation*

Along with these taxonomic, chemical, genomics, molecular and proteomic characterization; some chemical markers are also required to be identified using Thin Layer Chromatography(TLC), High-Performance Liquid Chromatography (HPLC), Capillary Electrophoresis (CE), and Mass Spectroscopy (MS), *etc.* All of

WHO   World Health Organization

CONSENT FOR PUBLICATION

Not applicable.

CONFLICT OF INTEREST

The author(s) confirms that there is no conflict of interest.

ACKNOWLEDGEMENTS

Declared none.

REFERENCES

[1]   World Health Organization. WHO remains firmly committed to the principles set out in the preamble to the Constitution [Internet] 2019.[cited 2019 Dec 20]. WHO remains firmly committed to the principles set out in the preamble to the Constitution.

[2]   Leitzmann C. Characteristics and Health Benefits of Phytochemicals. Forsch Komplement Med 2016; 23(2): 69-74.
[PMID: 27160996]

[3]   Botanical Drug Review [Internet] 2015.https://www.fda.gov/media/94221/download

[4]   WHO Expert Committee on Specifications for Pharmaceutical Preparations [Internet] 2018.https://apps.who.int/iris/bitstream/handle/10665/272452/9789241210195-eng.pdf?ua=1

[5]   Rates SM. Plants as source of drugs. Toxicon 2001; 39(5): 603-13.
[http://dx.doi.org/10.1016/S0041-0101(00)00154-9] [PMID: 11072038]

[6]   Sahoo N, Manchikanti P, Dey S. Herbal drugs: standards and regulation. Fitoterapia 2010; 81(6): 462-71. [Internet].
[http://dx.doi.org/10.1016/j.fitote.2010.02.001] [PMID: 20156530]

[7]   Astin JA. Why patients use alternative medicine: results of a national study. JAMA 1998; 279(19): 1548-53.
[http://dx.doi.org/10.1001/jama.279.19.1548] [PMID: 9605899]

[8]   WHO guidelines for assessing quality of herbal medicines with reference to contaminants and residues [Internet] 2007.http://apps.who.int/medicinedocs/index/assoc/s14878e/s14878e.pdf

[9]   Colalto C. Unpredictable Adverse Reactions to Herbal Products. J Drug Metabolism Toxicol 2012; 3(2): 2-4.

[10]   Mukherjee PK, Wahile A. Integrated approaches towards drug development from Ayurveda and other Indian system of medicines. J Ethnopharmacol 2006; 103(1): 25-35.
[http://dx.doi.org/10.1016/j.jep.2005.09.024] [PMID: 16271286]

[11]   National Policy on Traditional Medicine and Regulation of Herbal Medicines-Report of WHO Global Survey [Internet] Geneva 2005.https://apps.who.int/medicinedocs/en/d/Js7916e/

[12]   Wachtel-Galor S, Benzie IFF. Herbal Medicine-An Introduction to Its History, Usage, Regulation, Current Trends, and Research Needs. Herbal Medicine: Biomolecular and Clinical Aspect [Internet] II CRC PRess/Taylor & Francis 2011.https://www.ncbi.nlm.nih.gov/books/NBK92773/

[13]   Li JW-H, Vederas JC. Drug discovery and natural products: end of an era or an endless frontier? Science 2009; 325(5937): 161-5.

[http://dx.doi.org/10.1126/science.1168243] [PMID: 19589993]

[14]   Ardalan M-R, Rafieian-Kopaei M. Is the safety of herbal medicines for kidneys under question? J nephropharmacology 2013; 2(2): 11-2.

[15]   Elvin-Lewis M. Should we be concerned about herbal remedies. J Ethnopharmacol 2001; 75(2-3): 141-64.
[http://dx.doi.org/10.1016/S0378-8741(00)00394-9] [PMID: 11297844]

[16]   Cuzzolin L, Zaffani S, Benoni G. Safety implications regarding use of phytomedicines. Eur J Clin Pharmacol 2006; 62(1): 37-42.
[http://dx.doi.org/10.1007/s00228-005-0050-6] [PMID: 16328317]

[17]   WHO guidelines on safety monitoring of herbal medicines in pharmacovigilance systems [Internet] Geneva 2004.https://apps.who.int/medicinedocs/documents/s7148e/s7148e.pdf

[18]   Woolf AD. Safety evaluation and adverse events monitoring by poison control centers: a framework for herbs & dietary supplements. Clin Toxicol (Phila) 2006; 44(5): 617-22.
[http://dx.doi.org/10.1080/15563650600795578] [PMID: 16905504]

[19]   Vassilev ZP, Chu AF, Ruck B, Adams EH, Marcus SM. Evaluation of adverse drug reactions reported to a poison control center between 2000 and 2007. Am J Health Syst Pharm 2009; 66(5): 481-7.
[http://dx.doi.org/10.2146/ajhp080267] [PMID: 19233996]

[20]   Barnes J, Mills SY, Abbot NC, Willoughby M, Ernst E. Different standards for reporting ADRs to herbal remedies and conventional OTC medicines: face-to-face interviews with 515 users of herbal remedies. Br J Clin Pharmacol 1998; 45(5): 496-500.
[http://dx.doi.org/10.1046/j.1365-2125.1998.00715.x] [PMID: 9643624]

[21]   Xue J, Hao L, Peng F. Residues of 18 organochlorine pesticides in 30 traditional Chinese medicines. Chemosphere 2008; 71(6): 1051-5.
[http://dx.doi.org/10.1016/j.chemosphere.2007.11.014] [PMID: 18160094]

[22]   Saper RB, Kales SN, Paquin J, *et al.* Heavy metal content of ayurvedic herbal medicine products. JAMA 2004; 292(23): 2868-73.
[http://dx.doi.org/10.1001/jama.292.23.2868] [PMID: 15598918]

[23]   Saper RB, Phillips RS, Sehgal A, *et al.* Lead, mercury, and arsenic in US- and Indian-manufactured Ayurvedic medicines sold *via* the Internet. JAMA 2008; 300(8): 915-23.
[http://dx.doi.org/10.1001/jama.300.8.915] [PMID: 18728265]

[24]   Shaw D, Graeme L, Pierre D, Elizabeth W, Kelvin C. Pharmacovigilance of herbal medicine. J Ethnopharmacol 2012; 140(3): 513-8.
[http://dx.doi.org/10.1016/j.jep.2012.01.051] [PMID: 22342381]

[25]   Guidelines for the regulation of herbal medicines in the South-East Asia Region. WHO 2004.

[26]   General Guidelines for Methodologies on Research and Evaluation of Traditional Medicine World Health Organization [Internet] 2000.https://apps.who.int/medicinedocs/pdf/whozip42e/whozip42e.pdf

[27]   Herbal Preparation [Internet] [cited 2019 Dec 22]. https://www.ema.europa.eu/en/glossary/herbal-preparations

[28]   Folashade O, Omoregie H, Ochogu P. Standardization of herbal medicines -. Review 2012; 4(March): 101-12.

[29]   Herbal   Medicinal   Products :   Scientific   Guidelines   [Internet]   [cited   2019   Dec 9].https://www.ema.europa.eu/en/human-regulatory/researc--development/scientific-guidelines/multidisciplinary/herb-l-medicinal-products-scientific-guidelines#Clinical

[30]   Centre for Drug Evaluation and Research. Botanical Drug Development Guidance for Industry [Internet] 2016. https://www.fda.gov/media/93113/download

[31]   Guidelines For Inspection of GMP Compliance By ASU Drug Industry. New Delhi 2014.

[32]   WHO guidelines on good manufacturing practices (GMP) for herbal medicines [Internet] Geneva 2007.https://apps.who.int/medicinedocs/documents/s14215e/s14215e.pdf

[33]   Guideline on Specifications: Test Procedures and Acceptance Criteria For Herbal Substances, Herbal Preparations and Herbal Medicinal Products/Traditional Herbal Medicinal Products [Internet] London 2006.https://www.ema.europa.eu/en/documents/scientific-guideline/guideline-specifications-t-st-procedures-acceptance-criteria-herbal-substances-herbal-preparations/traditional-herbal--edicinal-products_en.pdf

[34]   Liang Y-Z, Xie P, Chan K. Quality control of herbal medicines. J Chromatogr B, Anal Technol Biomed life Sci 2004; 812(1-2): 53-70.

[35]   Research Guidelines for Evaluating the Safety and Efficacy of Herbal Medicines [Internet] 1993.https://apps.who.int/medicinedocs/en/d/Jh2946e/

[36]   Zhang K, Yan G, Zhang A, Wang X. Recent advances in pharmacokinetics approach for herbal medicine. Recent Adv 2017; 1(7): 28876-88.
[http://dx.doi.org/10.1039/C7RA02369C]

[37]   Yan R, Yang Y, Chen Y. Pharmacokinetics of Chinese medicines: strategies and perspectives. Chin Med 2018; 13: 24. [Internet].
[http://dx.doi.org/10.1186/s13020-018-0183-z] [PMID: 29743935]

[38]   Bansal G, Suthar N, Kaur J, Jain A. Stability testing of herbal drugs: Challenges, regulatory compliance and perspectives. Phytother Res 2016; 30(7): 1046-58.
[http://dx.doi.org/10.1002/ptr.5618] [PMID: 27073177]

[39]   Thakur L, Ghodasra U, Patel N, Dabhi M. Novel approaches for stability improvement in natural medicines. Pharmacogn Rev 2011; 5(9): 48-54.
[http://dx.doi.org/10.4103/0973-7847.79099] [PMID: 22096318]

[40]   Parveen A, Parveen B, Parveen R, Ahmad S. Challenges and guidelines for clinical trial of herbal drugs. J Pharm Bioallied Sci 2015; 7(4): 329-33.
[http://dx.doi.org/10.4103/0975-7406.168035] [PMID: 26681895]

CHAPTER 8

Quality Control of Herbal Medicinal Products

Javed Ahamad[1,*], Esra T. Anwer[2], Muath Sh. Mohammed Ameen[2], Jamia Firdous[3] and Nehal Mohsin[4]

[1] *Department of Pharmacognosy, Faculty of Pharmacy, Tishk International University, Kurdistan Region, Iraq*

[2] *Department of Pharmaceutics, Faculty of Pharmacy, Tishk International University, Kurdistan Region, Iraq*

[3] *Department of Pharmacy, Institute of Bio-Medical Education and Research, Mangalayatan University, Aligarh, India*

[4] *Department of Clinical Pharmacy, College of Pharmacy, Najran University, Kingdom of Saudi Arabia*

Abstract: The quality control of medicinal agents derived from natural sources is of paramount in ensuring safety and efficacy. The major hindrance in the acceptance of herbal medicines into modern medical practices is the lack of scientific and clinical data on the safety and efficacy of the herbal products. In general, there is a lack of strict guideline for quality control of herbal medicinal products used for the treatment of various human diseases. In recent years, due to enormous increased interest in herbal medicine, we need strict quality control parameters for safe and efficacious herbal medicine. Several quality control parameters (*e.g.* organoleptic, morphological, physico-chemical, chromatographic and toxic substances) are mentioned in Pharmacopoeias like Indian Pharmacopoeia (IP), British Herbal Pharmacopoeia (BHP), Ayurvedic Pharmacopoeia of India (API) and WHO guidelines *etc.* Chromatographic techniques, such as TLC, HPTLC, HPLC, GC-MS; and toxic substances such as aflatoxins, heavy metals, pesticide residues, microbial load determinations, are important parameters considered for quality control of herbal drugs. This book chapter provides a critical overview of different quality control parameters of herbal drug, which are necessary for compliance of regulatory guidelines of several developing and developed countries.

Keywords: HPTLC, Herbal Products, Pharmacopoeia, Quality Control, Standardization, WHO Guidelines.

* **Corresponding author Javed Ahamad:** Department of Pharmacognosy, Faculty of Pharmacy, Tishk International University, Kurdistan Region, Iraq; E-mails: jas.hamdard@gmail.com, javed.ahamad@tiu.edu.iq

Javed Ahmad and Javed Ahamad (Ed.)

1. INTRODUCTION

Standardization means adjusting the preparation of herbal drugs to a defined content of a constituent or group of substances having known therapeutic activity. Medicinal plants are widely used in herbal based drug formulations. While herbal medicinal products are often viewed as natural and healthy, they are not free from adverse effects. Such adverse effects of herbal drugs can occur due to adulteration, substitution, contamination, incorrect preparation and the most significant lack of standardization [1, 2]. The main criticism confronting the traditional medicine system is inadequate scientific validation and standards of plant material used by the manufacturer in herbal formulations. Quality control of herbal medicines is of paramount importance for its adoption in modern medical practices. The major problem with herbal medicine acceptance is the lack of data on herbal formulation on safety and efficacy. Standardization or quality control is of paramount importance to ensuring the therapeutic activity and safety of herbal drugs [3]. There are no standards for quality control of medicinal plants that are used in herbal formulation in most underdeveloped and developing countries. Quality control of herbal formulations is more complicated than synthetic formulations because of the complex nature of herbal drugs comprising several phytochemical compounds [4].

Usually, one or two most important chemical compounds chosen for analysis are used for quantitative analysis of bioactive phytochemicals in herbal formulations. Nonetheless, this type of determination does not give a complete picture of the formulation, as multiple constituents are usually responsible for their therapeutic effects [5]. Several chromatographic techniques, such as HPTLC, HPLC, GC, GC-MS, and LC-MS can be applied for this kind of documentation for quality control of herbal formulations and individual medicinal plants. For the purposes of chemical standardization and quality control of individual herbs and herbal formulations, chemical fingerprints obtained by chromatographic techniques are strongly recommended. Therefore, there is a strong need to promote standardization of quality parameters and formulations of important medicinal plants. WHO has emphasized the need to ensure quality control of medicinal plant products through the use of modern techniques and the application of appropriate standards. Several pharmacopoeias, including the United States Pharmacopoeia (USP), Indian Pharmacopoeia (IP), British Pharmacopoeia (BP), and British Herbal Pharmacopoeia (BHP), cover monographs and quality control tests for a few of the medicinal plants used in their respective countries [6]. This chapter of the book provides an overview of the various quality criteria applied to standardize herbal medicines.

2. THE NEED OF STANDARDIZATION

In general, adverse effects are thought to be less with herbal drugs compared to modern drugs, but reports on serious side effects indicate the need to develop effective marker-based standardization of herbal formulations [7]. Because of the lack of quality control measures on herbal formulations, people cannot make use of the benefits of these medicines. Because of scientific awareness, a scenario has been created for conducting research activities such as standardizing herbal formulations and developing scientific methods for large-scale production [8]. The idea of standardization is to establish consistent therapeutic effectiveness of batch-to-batch natural products [9 - 11].

3. METHODS OF STANDARDIZATION OF HERBAL MEDICINAL PRODUCTS

In recent years, due to enormous increased interest in herbal medicine, we need strict quality control parameters for safe and efficacious herbal medicine. Several quality control parameters such as organoleptic, morphological, physico-chemical, chromatographic (*e.g.* TLC, HPTLC, HPLC, GC-MS) and toxic substances (*e.g.* aflatoxins, heavy metals, pesticide residues, microbial load determinations) are mentioned in pharmacopoeias and WHO guidelines for ensuring safety and efficacy of herbal medicinal agents obtained from natural products [1, 12].

3.1. Botanical Parameters

3.1.1. Morphological Characters

Detailed study of morphological character may be useful in identifying various species of plants. A drug's morphological study includes the naked-eye visual appearance. Macroscopic analysis explores the following characters of the plant: size, shape, colour, taste, odour, fracture, *etc.* [6].

3.1.2. Powder Microscopy

Very small amounts of powdered drugs are taken on a slide and treated with gentle heating with HCl and chloral hydrate, and stained with phloroglucinol. After mounting with glycerin, observed under a compound microscope at suitable magnification. Powder microscopy helps in determining different types of tissues and cells present in plant materials such as phloem fibers, xylem vessels, tracheids, starch grains, *etc.*

3.2. Physico-Chemical Parameters

3.2.1. Extractive Values

Extraction methods are used to determine the desired bioactive compounds of any crude drugs. Extractive value with respect to specific solvents indicates the soluble matter of any drugs. As per WHO guidelines alcohol, water and hydro-alcohol soluble extractives are regularly used for the determination of extractive values of herbal drugs [6].

Cold extractive value: The powdered drug of approximately 4 g is macerated with various organic solvents of varying polarity (*e.g.* petroleum ether, chloroform, acetone, methanol, hydro-alcohol, and water) of volume 100 ml in a closed flask for 24 hours, frequently shaking at an interval of 6 hours and allowed to stand for 24 hours. It is rapidly filtered, and precautions are taken against solvent loss.

Hot extractive value: In Soxhlet apparatus, the powdered drug of about 4 g is packaged separately using 250 ml of different organic solvents (such as petroleum ether, chloroform, acetone, methanol, ethanol *etc.*). Each extract is evaporated to dryness, and with reference to air-dried material, constant extractive value is recorded.

Successive extractive value: The powdered drug of about 4 g is successively extracted in a Soxhlet apparatus with solvents such as petroleum ether, chloroform, acetone, methanol and hydro-alcohol, using the same drug for each solvent, respectively. The extract is concentrated by distilling off the solvent on a water bath or rota-evaporator and evaporating it to dryness [11, 12].

3.2.2. Ash Value

The residues that remain after incineration are the drug's total ash content, which simply represents the inorganic content of crude drugs. The drug's total ash is composed of physiological and non-physiological ash. Physiological ash is derived from plant tissues, whereas non-physiological ash is made up of residues of extraneous matter such as soil and sand. Ash value is a criterion for judging the identity and pureness of raw drugs. Acid-insoluble ash is also recommended for certain drugs, which is a part of total ash insoluble in dilute hydrochloric acid. Acid-insoluble ash is used to determine dirt and sands, which are adhered to raw drugs [11].

Total ash: The total ash is designed to measure the total amount of material remaining after ignition. Accurately weighed (about 2-3 g) air dried crude drug was placed in the tared platinum or silica dish and was incinerated at a temperature not exceeding 450 °C until free from carbon, cooled and weighed to get the total ash content.

Acid insoluble ash: Acid insoluble ash is the residue obtained after boiling the total ash with diluted hydrochloric acid (10% in distilled water) and igniting the remaining insoluble matter. This measures the amount of silica present, especially as sand and siliceous earth. Ash was boiled with 25 ml of hydrochloric acid for 5 minutes. The insoluble matter was collected on ash less filter paper, washed with hot water and ignited at a temperature not exceeding 450 °C to a constant weigh.

Water soluble ash: Water soluble ash is the difference in weight between the total ash and the residue after treatment with water. It is a good indicator of either previous extraction of water-soluble salts in the drug or incorrect preparation. Ash was dissolved in distilled water and the insoluble part collected on an ash less filter paper and was ignited at 450 °C to a constant weight. By subtracting the weight of insoluble part from that of ash, the weight of the soluble part of ash was obtained.

3.2.3. Loss on Drying

Loss on drying is employed in many official books, including BP and USP, as a quality control parameter. The weight loss in tested samples of plant drugs, primarily due to water and a small amount of other volatile materials, also contributes to the weight loss. For plant drugs such as senna, digitalis, aloes, *etc.* that contain little volatile material, direct drying (100-105 °C) to constant weight can be employed. Crude drugs containing considerable amounts of volatile oil such as balsams, cardamom, clove, peppermint, *etc.* should be dried either by toluene distillation process or spread over a thin layer of paper, accompanied by drying over phosphorus pentoxide in desiccator [1, 11].

3.2.4. Foreign Organic Matter

The parts of the plants other than those named in the crude drug definition and description are defined as foreign organic matter. In the crude drugs monograph the maximum limit for foreign organic matter is defined. If the foreign matter exceeds the limits specified in pharmacopoeias, the drug should be discarded. Accurately measured samples of synthetic drugs (100-500 g) are taken and distributed over the paper in a thin layer. The sample removes foreign matter or unwanted plant materials, and the sample is again weighed to know the percentage of foreign matter present [1, 12].

3.2.5. Swelling Index

Several medicinal plants materials have swelling properties such as isapgol, and commonly used as bulk laxatives. The swelling index of such plant materials was determined by taking 1 g of drug material in 25 ml of water in stoppered measuring cylinder for 3 hours [11].

3.2.6. Foaming Index

Several crude drugs contain saponins that form foams when shaken by aqueous solutions. These foaming properties of drug-containing saponin are measured as an index of foaming, and represent a parameter of quality control. Around 1 gm of coarse powder of plant material is taken in 500 ml conical flask containing 100 ml of boiling water for measurement of the foaming index. Further, the drug is boiled at a moderate temperature for 30 minutes. The flask is then cooled and filtered into a measuring cylinder of up to 100 ml, and finally the foaming index is measured [11].

3.2.7. Fat Content

Fat content for those crude drugs that contain fixed oils and lipids is usually determined. In Soxhlet apparatus, about 4 g of the powdered crude drug is extracted with anhydrous ether for 6 hours in order to determine the fat content of plant materials, and then extract is filtered into a clean and dry weighed flask. At 105 °C, the solvent is evaporated and dried up to constant weight.

3.2.8. Resin Content

For such drugs, the resin content is determined, which contains considerable quantities of resins such as ginger, capsicum, *etc*. For resin content determination, approximately 4 g of crude drug is refluxed with non-polar solvent such as acetone (3×200 ml) for 6 hours to exhaust resin content.

The extract obtained is suspended in water and transferred to the funnel separation and extracted with ether (3×200 ml) to extract all resins. The ether extract is evaporated and dried over anhydrous sodium sulphate, and the final yield is calculated using the formula below [6].

$$\% \text{ Resin content } = \frac{\text{Weight of extract} \times 100}{\text{Weight of drug}}$$

3.2.9. Total Flavonoid Content

Flavonoids are secondary plant metabolites with enormous pharmacological activity. Quercetin is used for determining the total flavonoids in plant medicinal products. The method for determining total flavonoid is briefly described as:

Reagents: $AlCl_3$ (0.1 g/ml) and CH_3COONa (1M) are prepared, prepared dilution for quercetin (standard) from 10 µg/ml to 100 µg/ml.

Preparation of samples: Take approximately 10 mg/ml solution of the test sample in methanol and add 0.5 ml of the test sample in 1.5 ml of methanol. To this, 0.1 ml of $AlCl_3$, 0.1 ml of CH_3COONa and 2.8 ml of distilled water were added and kept for 30 minutes. The absorbance is measured at 415 nm and values are recorded.

Standard curve preparation: Similarly, standard quercetin dilutions are prepared and absorbance recorded.

Preparation of blank solution: in blank solutions test and standard is replaced with methanol.

Finally, the calibration curve is prepared from standard quercetin dilutions and then the total flavonoid content is calculated using the standard calibration curve in the test sample [13].

Preparation of standard curve: Similarly, standard dilutions of quercetin solution are prepared and absorbance is recorded.

3.2.10. Total Phenolic Content

Briefly, total phenolic content is determined as: reagents: 10 percent Folin-Ciocalteu reagent, Na_2CO_3 (1 M) is prepared in distilled water and standard gallic acid stack solution (1 mg/ml) in methanol.

Preparation of test samples: Approximately, 100 mg of powdered crude drug was dissolved and filtered in 10 ml of methanol, followed by the addition of 5 ml 10% Folin-Ciocalteu reagent and 4 ml of Na_2CO_3. After 15 minutes, the absorbance is measured at 765 nm, and values are recorded.

Preparation of standard curve: Similarly, standard solution was prepared and the absorbance of serial dilutions of standard solution is recorded.

Preparation of blank solution: in blank solutions test and standard is replaced with methanol.

Finally, the calibration curve was prepared from standard gallic acid dilutions and total phenolic content is calculated using the standard calibration curve in the test sample [13].

3.3. General Quality Parameters

3.3.1. Fluorescence Analysis

Powdered plant materials, when visualized under daylight and UV-visible light after treatment with certain chemicals, show fluorescence and these are characteristic features for individual drugs. The powdered material (about 40 mesh) is treated with chemical reagents such as sodium hydroxide, hydrochloric acid, nitric acid, ferric chloride, *etc.* to assess the fluorescence activity of synthetic drugs and then visualize in daylight and UV light (254 and 366 nm) [14 - 16].

3.3.2. Powdered Drug Reaction with Chemical Reagents

Upon treatment with certain chemical reagents such as sodium hydroxide, picric acid, acetic acid, hydrochloric acid, nitric acid, iodine *etc.*, the action of powdered crude drugs creates specific colors which can be observed under a microscope. It is a good indicator of plant materials in the deciding phytochemical class of plant materials [17].

3.4. Phytochemical Screening

These are simple chemical tests that are performed to know the chemical class of crude drugs such as alkaloids, glycosides, carbohydrates, flavonoids, tannins, flavonoids, resins and terpenes, *etc.* In order to perform these phytochemical screening, first crude drugs are extracted with appropriate solvents and processed accordingly to have a proper amount of secondary metabolites. The specific methods for each class of secondary metabolites are given in several Pharmacognosy text books [18 - 21].

3.5. Determination of Toxic Residues

Toxic residues in herbal formulation are becoming a major cause of cancer, and about 30% of cancers are caused by toxic foods. Toxic residues in crude herbal drugs and finished formulations arise as a result of the application of pesticides during cultivation of medicinal crops and the use of these pesticides during storage. Some countries applied guidelines for controlling the levels of pesticides in both crude drugs and finished herbal formulations.

3.5.1. Pesticide Residues

Pesticide levels in crude drugs and finished herbal formulation can be determined by gas chromatography and gas chromatography mass spectroscopy.

For quantification of each pesticide, standard pesticide is co-injected in GC/MS.

If the pesticide to which the plant material has been exposed is known or can be identified by suitable means, an established method for the determination of that particular pesticide residue should be used. Pesticide residues may be reduced by the use of organic forming or by the use of infusions of the dried plant materials and by the extraction of useful plant constituents [1].

3.5.2. Aflatoxin Residue

Aflatoxins are toxic contaminants present in crude herbal drugs that cause severe complications in humans and animals. Aflatoxins such as B_1, B_2, G_1 and G_2 should be determined in herbal formulation before marketing. Generally, thin layer chromatography is used for the determination of aflatoxins in herbal drugs. Due to the advancement of quantitative techniques such as high performance thin layer chromatography (HPTLC), now quantitative determination of aflatoxins became easy and fast. For the determination of aflatoxins by the TLC method, standard aflatoxins solutions are run along with unknown test samples of plant materials or finished herbal formulations and spots are compared. If spots in the test sample match with the standard one, then qualitatively, we can determine the type of aflatoxins in the test sample. For the quantitative determination of aflatoxins by HPTLC method, serial dilutions of standard aflatoxins are prepared and from these solutions standard curve is prepared and finally the concentration of test samples is obtained from standard curve [1].

3.5.3. Microbial Load

Medicinal plant products usually contain a large number of microbes such as bacteria and moulds, which are mostly field-based. Current herbal product processing, storage, and manufacturing practices also cause additional contamination and microbial growth. The presence of these microbes causes serious risks to human health and should be determined in crude and finished herbal medicines by suitable means. British Pharmacopoeia (BP) requires a number of herbal drugs free from *Escherichia coli* (for *e.g.* Acacia, agar, starch, sterculia, tragacanth, powdered digitalis) and *Salmonella* (*e.g.* alginic acid, cochineal, guar, tragacanth). The upper limits for the total viable aerobic count, commonly 10^3, 10^4 microorganism g^{-1}, are being increasingly applied to crude drugs [22, 23].

3.5.4. Heavy Metal Toxicity

Medicinal plants and herbal formulations are sometimes contaminated with heavy metals such as lead, mercury, zinc, cadmium and arsenic. These heavy metals cause serious health hazards in humans and should be controlled in finished herbal formulations. The official limits (parts per million) of such heavy metals in medicinal plants and finished herbal medicines should be determined and kept within limits. For the determination of heavy metals, atomic absorption spectroscopy (AAS) is used [1, 6]. Natural products or herbal drugs should comply with the WHO guidelines and the Pharmacopoeial monograph on herbal drugs with respect to heavy metal content.

3.6. Chromatographic Evaluation of Herbal Medicinal Products

2.6.1. Thin Layer Chromatography and R_F Values

Thin layer chromatography is a simple, fast and reliable method of analyzing herbal drugs qualitatively and semi-quantitatively. Several pharmacopoeias have included TLC as reference method for herbal drug analysis. In this method, test plant samples in the form of extract in suitable solvents are run along with the standard plant samples [1]. The test plant sample is compared with the standard plant based on the number and color of TLC spots. If the number and color of the spots in both are the same, the test sample will pass otherwise it would fail. R_F values determined for a compound under specific conditions are characteristic and can be used as an aid to phytocompound identification [20, 24].

3.6.2. High Performance Thin Layer Chromatography (HPTLC)

High performance thin layer chromatography (HPTLC) is the most widely used analytical tools for herbal industries. HPTLC is a planer chromatography, which became superior to TLC as a powerful analytical technique with high separation, performance and reproducibility. It provides the means for flexible screening procedures, qualitative analysis and quantitative determination [25, 26]. HPTLC is a flexible and cost effective alternative HPLC that allows post chromatographic derivatization. HPTLC technique is especially suitable for comparison of samples based on finger printing and it has become a cost and time effective alternative to HPLC [27]. Nowadays, HPTLC technique is routinely used for quality control of herbal products [28 - 30].

3.6.3. High Pressure Liquid Chromatography (HPLC)

High-pressure liquid chromatography (HPLC) is the most common technique used for the analysis of herbal products, synthetic drugs, cosmetics and food products. HPLC is a popular method for the identification and quantification of herbal products because it is easy to learn and use, moreover, it is not limited by the volatility or stability of the sample compound [31]. Liquid chromatography coupled with a mass spectrometer is the method of choice in developed countries for quantitative analysis of synthetic and herbal formulations. This method provides accurate, reliable, fast and reproducible results [1].

3.6.4. Gas Chromatography-Mass Spectrometry (GC-MS)

Gas chromatography-mass spectrometry (GC-MS) technique is fast and has a high power of resolution and high sensitivity. GC-MS now days become a very good technique for the identification and characterization of volatile or essential oil [32]. GC-MS is a hyphenated analytical technique. As the name implies, it is actually two techniques that are combined to form a single method of analyzing mixtures of chemical compounds. Gas chromatography separates the components of a mixture and mass spectroscopy characterizes each of the components individually. By combining the two techniques, an analytical chemist can both qualitatively and quantitatively analyze samples containing essential oils, fixed oils, amino acids and peptides *etc*. GC-MS is nowadays included as a quality control parameter in several pharmacopoeias like Ayurvedic Pharmacopoeia of India (API), ICMR monographs for medicinal plants containing essential oils [33 - 35].

3.6.5. Liquid Chromatography-Mass Spectrometry (LC-MS)

Mass spectroscopy is the most specific technique for correct identification of synthetic as well as natural compounds. In this technique, molecular weight and fragmentation pattern of any chemical compound is determined exactly. When mass spectroscopy is coupled with liquid chromatography, the separation and identification become very fast and reliable. That is why in today's scenario, LC-MS becomes the method of choice for analysis and identification of phytochemicals. The continuous separation and quantification process can be accomplished by coupling the liquid chromatography (LC) techniques with mass spectrometry (MS). That is why LC is now paired with MS to identify and characterize natural compounds expeditiously and efficiently [36, 37]. Because of its speed and accuracy in assessing molecular mass, mass spectrometry is an important method for the structural assessment of natural products. Mass spectroscopy just requires samples in micrograms to be evaluated and gives reliable and reproducible results. Mass spectrometry is also commonly used to evaluate substances with the previously reported mass spectrum, and analyze new unknown compounds as well. The catalogue of the identified compounds is measured and compared for an already known compound with the spectrum of the compound in question. Samples are ionized in mass spectroscopy by allowing them to travel through an analyser where they are detected by the mass to charge ratio. The vapor of the sample is made to disperse in the low pressure system of the mass spectrometer, which ionizes the compound with sufficient energy and allows it to be fragmented. This allows positive ions to be produced that are stimulated by the applied magnetic field and are moving according to the mass to charge ratio [38]. LC-MS is utilized both in quantitative analysis and also in structural characterization of chemical compounds alongwith other spectroscopic techniques such as UV, IR and NMR [39].

CONCLUDING REMARKS

The quality control is an important step in ensuring the safety and efficacy of natural or herbal products. In recent years, due to enormous increased interest in herbal medicine, we need strict quality control parameters for safe and efficacious herbal medicine. Several quality control parameters *e.g.*, organoleptic, morphological, physico-chemical, chromatographic and toxic substances are mentioned in several pharmacopoeias and WHO guidelines. Chromatographic techniques, such as TLC, HPTLC, HPLC, GC-MS and toxic substances such as aflatoxins, heavy metals, pesticide residues, microbial load determinations, are important parameters considered for quality control of herbal drugs. Safety, purity and efficacy of herbal medicines are only possible if herbal products are manufactured under GMP and good quality parameters followed for the crude drugs as well as finished products.

ABBREVIATIONS

AAS   Atomic Absorption Spectrometer

API   Ayurvedic Pharmacopoeia of India

BP   British Pharmacopoeia

BHP   British Herbal Pharmacopoeia

GC-MS   Gas chromatography Mass spectrometry

GMP   Good Manufacturing practice

HPTLC   High performance thin layer chromatography

HPLC   High performance liquid chromatography

IP   Indian Pharmacopoeia

TLC   Thin layer chromatography

WHO   World health organization

CONSENT FOR PUBLICATION

Not applicable.

CONFLICT OF INTEREST

The author(s) confirms that there is no conflict of interest.

ACKNOWLEDGEMENTS

Declared none.

REFERENCES

[1]   Mukherjee PK. Quality control of Herbal Drugs. 1st ed., Delhi: Business Horizons Pharmaceutical Publishers 2002.

[2]   Lau AJ, Holmes MJ, Wood SO, Koh HL. Analysis of adulterants in a traditional herbal medicinal products using liquid chromatography-mass spectrometry. J Pharm Biomed Anal 2003; 31: 401-6.
[http://dx.doi.org/10.1016/S0731-7085(02)00637-4] [PMID: 12609680]

[3]   Gogtay NJ, Bhatt HA, Dalvi SS, Kshirsagar NA. The use and safety of non-allopathic Indian medicines. Drug Saf 2002; 25(14): 1005-19.
[http://dx.doi.org/10.2165/00002018-200225140-00003] [PMID: 12408732]

[4]   Xie Y, Jiang ZH, Zhou H, *et al.* Combinative method using HPLC quantitative and qualitative analyses for quality consistency assessment of a herbal medicinal preparation. J Pharm Biomed Anal 2007; 43(1): 204-12.
[http://dx.doi.org/10.1016/j.jpba.2006.07.008] [PMID: 16920317]

[5]   Yan XJ, Zhou JJ, Xie GR, Milne GWA. Traditional Chinese medicines: molecular structures, natural sources and applications. Aldershot: Ashgate 1999.

[6]   Quality control methods for medicinal plant material. Geneva: World Health Organization 1998; pp. 8-78.

[7]   Sahoo N, Manchikanti P, Dey S. Herbal drugs: standards and regulation. Fitoterapia 2010; 81(6): 462-71.
[http://dx.doi.org/10.1016/j.fitote.2010.02.001] [PMID: 20156530]

[8]   Meena R, Meena AK, Khan SA, Mageswari S. Evaluation of a Unani compound formulation *Majoon-e-Sandal*. Int J Pharm Sci Res 2010; 1(5): 238-42.

[9]   Chaudhari RD. Herbal drug Industry, A practical approach to industrial pharmacognosy. New Delhi: Eastern Publishers 1996; pp. 45-78.

[10]   Gupta AK. Quality Standards of Indian Medicinal Plants. 2003.

[11]   Ahamad J, Mir SR, Naquvi KJ. Preliminary pharmacognostical standardization of aerial parts of *Artemisia absinthium* Linn. Int Res J Pharm 2012; 3(1): 217-20. a

[12]   Ahamad J, Mir SR, Naquvi KJ. Development of quality standards of *Berberis aristata* stem bark. Int Res J Pharm 2012; 3(2): 184-8. b

[13]   Pourmorad F, Hosseinimehr SJ, Shahabimajd N. Antioxidant activity, phenol and flavonoid contents of some selected Iranian medicinal plants. Afr J Biotechnol 2006; 5(11): 1142-5.

[14]   Chase CR Jr, Pratt R. Fluorescence of powdered vegetable drugs with particular reference to development of a system of identification. J Am Pharm Assoc Am Pharm Assoc 1949; 38(6): 324-31.
[http://dx.doi.org/10.1002/jps.3030380612] [PMID: 18145471]

[15]   Kokoshi CJ, Kokoski RJ, Sharma PJ. Fluorescence of powdered vegetable drugs under UV radiation. J Am Pharm Assoc 1958; 47: 715-7.
[http://dx.doi.org/10.1002/jps.3030471010]

[16]   Sama V, Swamy MM, Vijayalakshm S, Reddy YSR, Suresh B. Pharmacognostical observation on *Sidarhomboidea*: a report. Indian Drugs 1994; 3(9): 421-9.

[17]   Pharmacopoeial Standards for Ayurvedic formulation Central council for research in Ayerveda and Siddha, Ministry of Health and Family Welfare. Govt. of India, New Delhi.

[18]   Ali M. Text Book of Pharmacognosy. 2003.

[19]   Harborne JB. Phytochemical methods-A guide to modern technique of plant analysis. 3rd ed. London: Chapman and Hall 1998; pp. 109-45.

[20]   Trease GE, Evans WC. Pharmacognosy. 16th ed., London: Bailliere Tindall 2009.

[21]   Farnsworth NR. Biological and phytochemical screening of plants. J Pharm Sci 1966; 55(3): 225-76.
[http://dx.doi.org/10.1002/jps.2600550302] [PMID: 5335471]

[22]   Quality control methods for Medicinal plant materials. Geneva 1998.

[23]   Indian Pharmacopoeia Ministry of Health and Family Welfare, Controller of Publication, Govt of India, New Delhi.

[24]   Wagner H, Bladt S, Zgainsk EM. Plant drug Analysis: A thin layer chromatography Atlas. Berlin: Springer, Verlag 1984.
[http://dx.doi.org/10.1007/978-3-662-02398-3]

[25]   Ahamad J, Hassan N, Amin S, Mir SR. Development and validation of HPTLC-densitometry method for the quantification of swertiamarin in traditional bitters and formulations. J Planar Chromatogr Mod TLC 2015; 28(1): 61-8.
[http://dx.doi.org/10.1556/JPC.28.2015.1.10]

[26]   Ahamad J, Amin S, Mir SR. Simultaneous quantification of gymnemic acid and charantin using validated HPTLC densitometric method. J Chromatogr Sci 2014; 53(7): 1203-9.
[http://dx.doi.org/10.1093/chromsci/bmu166] [PMID: 25523465]

[27]   Sethi PD. HPTLC: High Performance Thin Layer Chromatography. New Delhi, India: CBS Publishers and Distributors 1996.

[28]   Hassan N, Ahamad J, Amin S, Mir SR. Rapid preparative isolation of erythrocentaurin from *Enicostemma littorale* by medium pressure liquid chromatography, its estimation by a validated HPTLC densitometric method and α-amylase inhibitory activity. J Sep Sci 2015; 38(4): 592-8.
       [http://dx.doi.org/10.1002/jssc.201401030] [PMID: 25504557]

[29]   Naquvi KJ, Ansari SH, Ahamad J. Development and validation of HPTLC method for estimation of imperatorin in anti-obesity polyherbal formulation, *Safoof-e-Muhazzil* and its ingredients. Asian J Tradit Med 2014; 9(2): 34-44. a

[30]   Naquvi KJ, Ansari SH, Ali M, Ahamad J. Development and validation of HPTLC densitometric method for simultaneous estimation of quercetin and kaempferol in herbal extracts and polyherbal formulation. Drug Discov Develop 2014; 1(2): 94-102. b

[31]   Ahamad J, Amin S, Mir SR. Development and validation of HPLC-UV method for estimation of swertiamarin in *Enicostemma littorale*. J Pharm Biomed Sci 2014; 1: 9-16.

[32]   Ahamad J, Uthirapathy S, Ameen MSM, Anwer ET. Essential oil composition and antidiabetic, anticancer activity of Rosmarinus officinalis L leaves from Erbil. Iraq: J Essent Oil Bear Plants 2019.
       [http://dx.doi.org/10.1080/0972060X.2019.1689179]

[33]   Hamad KJ, Al-Shaheen SJA, Kaskoos RA, Javed A, Jameel M, Mir SR. Essential oil composition and antioxidant activity of *Lavandula angustifolia* from Iraq. Int Res J Pharm 2013; 4(4): 117-20.

[34]   Naquvi KJ, Ahamad J, Ali M, Ansari SH, Salma A. Analysis of essential oil of *Origanum vulgare* Linn by GC and GC-MS. J Glob Trends Pharm Sci 2018; 9(3): 5786-91.

[35]   Uthirapathy S, Ahamad J. Phytochemical analysis of different fractions of *Terminalia arjuna* bark by GC-MS. Int Res J Pharm 2019; 10(1): 42-8.
       [http://dx.doi.org/10.7897/2230-8407.10018]

[36]   Johnson D, Orlando R. Optimization of data-dependent parameters for LC-MS/MS protein identification. J Biomol Tech 2011; 22 (Suppl.): S57-8.

[37]   Shevchenko A, Jensen ON, Podtelejnikov AV, *et al.* Linking genome and proteome by mass spectrometry: large-scale identification of yeast proteins from two dimensional gels. Proc Natl Acad Sci USA 1996; 93(25): 14440-5.
       [http://dx.doi.org/10.1073/pnas.93.25.14440] [PMID: 8962070]

[38]   Matros A, Kaspar S, Witzel K, Mock HP. Recent progress in liquid chromatography-based separation and label-free quantitative plant proteomics. Phytochemistry 2011; 72(10): 963-74.
       [http://dx.doi.org/10.1016/j.phytochem.2010.11.009] [PMID: 21176926]

[39]   Delahunty C, Yates JR III. Protein identification using 2D-LC-MS/MS. Methods 2005; 35(3): 248-55.
       [http://dx.doi.org/10.1016/j.ymeth.2004.08.016] [PMID: 15722221]

CHAPTER 9

Regulatory perspectives of Herbal Medicinal Products

Faraat Ali[1,*], Shaik Khasimbi[2], Kamna Sharma[3], Manisha Trivedi[4], Asad Ali[5] and Javed Ahmad[6,*]

[1] *Laboratory Services, Botswana Medicines Regulatory Authority, Plot 112 International Finance Park, Gaborone, Botswana*

[2] *Department of Pharmaceutical Chemistry, Delhi Institute of Pharmaceutical Sciences and Research (DIPSAR), Mehrauli-Badarpur Road, Push Vihar, Sector-3, New Delhi, 110017, India*

[3] *Department of Pharmaceutical Analysis, Indo-Soviet Friendship College of Pharmacy, Moga, Punjab, India*

[4] *NIMS University, Jaipur, Rajasthan, India*

[5] *Department of Chemistry, School of Chemical and Life Sciences, Jamia Hamdard University, New Delhi, India*

[6] *Department of Pharmaceutics, College of Pharmacy, Najran University, KSA*

Abstract: Quality control of medicinal agents derived from natural sources is paramount in ensuring safety and efficacy. In the modern medical practice, the major obstacles for the acceptance of herbal medicines are the lack of scientific and clinical data on safety, quality and efficacy in herbal products. In general, there is no quality control of medicinal products in many countries. Strict regulatory guidelines on herbal products are followed only in few countries like Canada, Europe, Australia, the USA, and Japan. In recent years, due to the enormous increased interest in herbal medicines, we need strict regulatory guidelines to ensure safety and efficacy of herbal medicine. The regulatory guidelines should focus mainly on laws related to the registration of herbal medicines for manufacturing and marketing. This book chapter will provide a comprehensive overview of a regulatory guidelines, required for manufacturing and marketing of herbal medicines in regulated, semi-regulated and unregulated markets. This book chapter also comprises discussion over global need of harmonization of regulatory guidelines to ensure safe and effective use of herbal medicines.

Keywords: Efficacy, Herbal Medicines, Harmonization, Pharmacopoeia, Regulatory Agency, Safety.

* **Corresponding author Faraat Ali and Javed Ahmad:** Laboratory Services, Botswana Medicines Regulatory Authority (BoMRA), Gaborone, Botswana and Department of Pharmaceutics, College of Pharmacy, Najran University, KSA; E-mails: FRHTL6@gmail.com & jahmad18@gmail.com

1. INTRODUCTION

Generally, it is to be believed that the risks associated with herbal drugs are minimal, but reports on serious adverse effects show the need for strict regulatory guidelines. The drug discovery on the basis of the natural product has experienced indefinite number of challenges, such as identification, availability of bioactive ingredients, *etc*. Although diverse approach including novel and potential therapeutic agents modulating cell signaling cascades are popular, for the drug discovery of natural products from medicinal plants [1]. The drug discovery of medicinal plants have played an important role in curing cancer (*e.g.* Vincristine, Vinblastine, Paclitaxel, Docetaxel, *etc*.) and malaria (*e.g.* Quinine, Artemisinin). The drug discovery from plants today is an expensive and time-consuming process, it requires a team efforts consisting of experts from different disciplines, such as pharmacognosists, pharmacologists, medicinal chemist and pharmaceutists. The trend today, especially in an industrial setting, is to seek bioactive phytochemicals that will serve as a lead compound in drug discovery and used for synthetic or semi-synthetic drug development, to make sure patent protection [2]. Newman and Cragg, reported that totally 1562 new drugs approved during 1981 to 2014, out of which natural products (04%; N), natural product derivatives (21%; ND), synthetic drugs with natural-derived pharmacophores (10%; S*/NM), and synthetic drugs designed based on knowledge gained from a natural product (11%; S/NM). The above reports suggested that the natural products are important source, hence involved in the new drug development as natural drugs or semi-synthetic drugs [3]. The plants considered as equal or superior in the drug discovery because of their chemical diversity and human friendly nature based on their long history of use for consumption.

The natural medicinal product has played an important role to give basic healthcare requirements of the population. The World Health Organization (WHO) has defined natural medicine along with allopathic medicines for improvement and prevention of illness. In Asian countries such as Korea, China, India and Japan, the natural medicinal plants plays a vital role in curing different diseases. However, each country has its own unique traditional systems such as the traditional Indian medicine (TIM), traditional Korean medicine (TKM), traditional Chinese medicine (TCM) and traditional Japanese medicine (TJM). In India, there are seven well-known different systems of medicines *i.e.* Ayurveda, Yoga, Siddha System of Medicine (SSM), Unani Medical System (UMS), Naturopathy, Homoeopathy, and Amchi Medical System (AMS) [4 - 7]. The plant materials used in many herbal medicinal products manufactured for general retail sale are not standardized. The quality control system in the development for various herbal preparations is much more difficult than for synthetic drugs because of the chemical complexity of their ingredients. As herbal preparations are composed of 100 unique or species-specific compounds, various difficulties are completely characterized by all these compounds. Thus, there is a pertaining need in promoting standardization for various quality parameters in medicinal plants and formulations. WHO emphasized the need to ensure quality control of herbal plant products by using modern techniques and applying suitable standards [8]. Several pharmacopoeias including United States Pharmacopoeia (USP), Indian Pharmacopoeia (IP), British Pharmacopoeia (BP), and British Herbal Pharmacopoeia (BHP) covers monographs and quality control tests for few of the medicinal plants used in the respective countries (Table 1).

Table 1. Regional Regulating Bodies in different countries.

Countries	Regulatory Bodies
India	Ayurveda, Yoga and Naturopathy, Unani, Siddha and Homoeopathy (AYUSH)
Australia	Therapeutic Goods Administration (TGA)
Canada	Health Canada
China	State Food and Drug Administration
Europe	European Medicine Agency (EMA)
Malaysia	National Pharmaceutical Control Bureau
USA	United States Food and Drug Administration (USFDA)
Singapore	Health Science Authority (HSA)
South Korea	Korean Food and Drug Administration (KFDA)
Saudi Arabia	Saudi Food and Drug Authority (SFDA)
Japan	Pharmaceutical and Medical devices Agency (PMDA)
Indonesia	National Agency of Drug and food control (NADFC)
Brazil	Agencia Nacional de Vigilancia Sanitaria (ANVISA)
South Africa	South African Health Products Regulatory Agency (SAHPRA)
New Zealand	New Zealand Medicine and Medical Devices Safety Authority
United Kingdom	Medicines and Healthcare Products Regulatory agency ((MHRA)
Tanzania	Tanzania Food and Drug Administration (TFDA)
Botswana	Botswana Medicine Regulatory Authority (BoMRA)

In the recent years traditional medicines has been regulated by different authorities of the respective countries to ensure the safety and efficacy of these drugs [9]. Various regulatory authorities have designed the guidance for the effective and safe use of medicines to avoid the adverse effect and to improve healthcare. WHO has proposed various guidelines for the herbal products that act as a reference standard for various countries to keep up the quality and safety of these medicinal products. WHO has launched "WHO traditional medicine strategies for 2014-2023" to promote the use of traditional medicines for healthcare and to improve the quality, effectiveness and safety of such medicine on humans and animals [10]. This book chapter provides a comprehensive overview of regulatory guidance that act as mandate for manufacturing and marketing of traditional medicine in regulated, semi-regulated and unregulated markets. This book chapter also encompasses the global need for harmonization of regulatory guidance on herbal medicine for ensuring safety and efficacy.

2. NEED AND CHALLENGES IN HERBAL PRODUCT REGULATIONS

Understanding the chronological development of herbal pharmaceutical industry will give an insight of regulatory network and the regulators. Currently in place and required for healthy growth of herbal medicine market (Fig. **1**) [11 - 13].

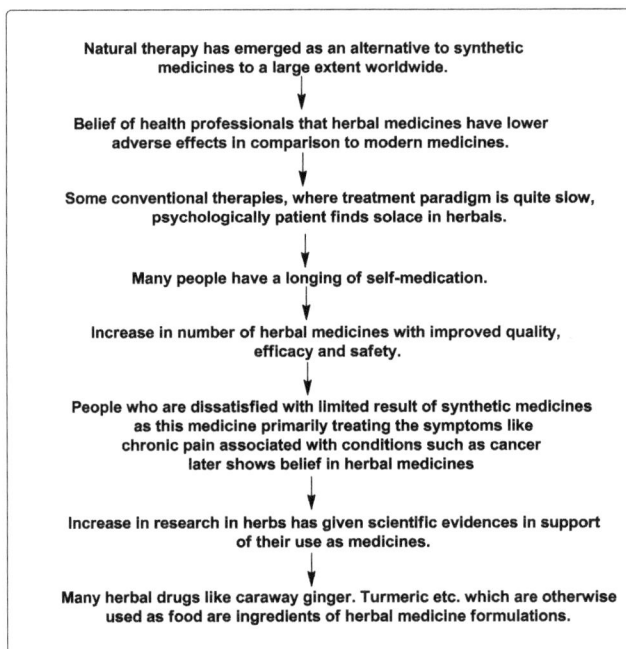

Fig. (1). The Growth of herbal medicine is the most important factors are responsible for worldwide in Pharma industry.

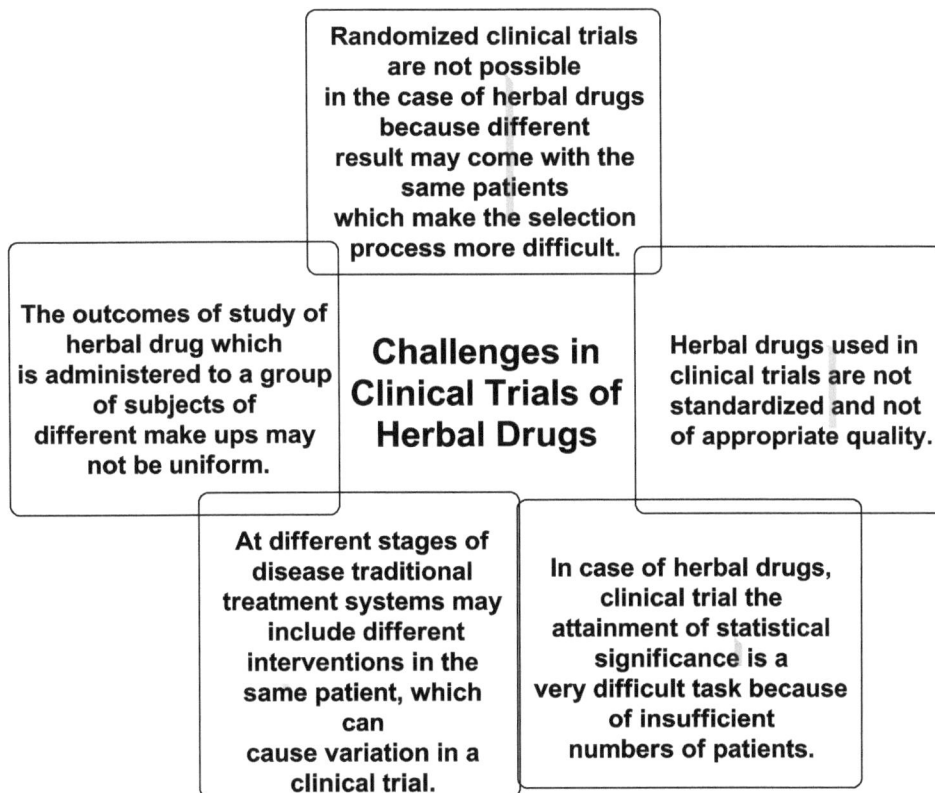

Fig. (2). The Herbal drugs with different challenges in clinical trials.

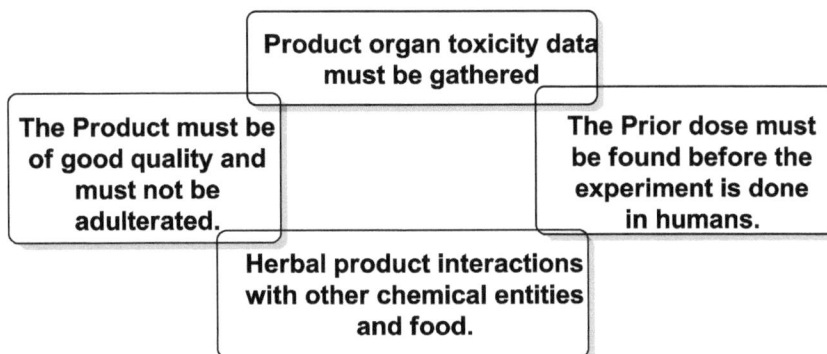

Fig. (3). Herbal products on ethical considerations in clinical trials.

3. INTERNATIONAL REGULATORY SCENARIO

In present scenario herbal preparations vary around the world, in some countries these preparations follow legislative criteria while others with no legislative regulations [14]. The regulatory bodies are special licensing systems which need to work with health authorities for development of various constituents. The regulatory bodies analyze proofs for safety and quality before marketing. Obliging license was reported for adverse reactions within a post-marketing system [15] (Fig. **4**).

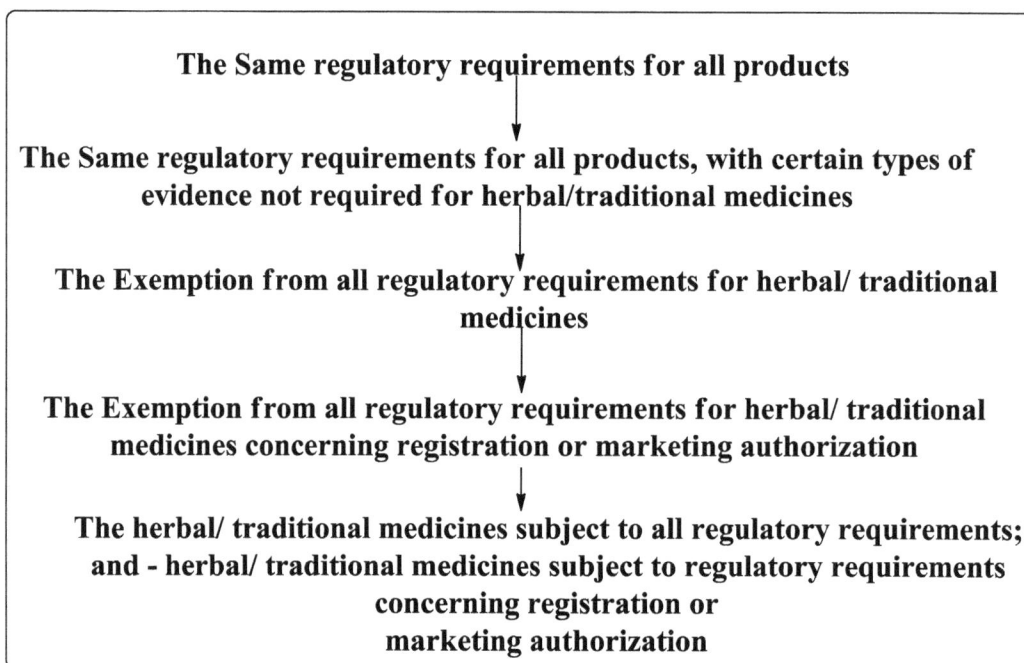

The Same regulatory requirements for all products

↓

The Same regulatory requirements for all products, with certain types of evidence not required for herbal/traditional medicines

↓

The Exemption from all regulatory requirements for herbal/ traditional medicines

↓

The Exemption from all regulatory requirements for herbal/ traditional medicines concerning registration or marketing authorization

↓

The herbal/ traditional medicines subject to all regulatory requirements; and - herbal/ traditional medicines subject to regulatory requirements concerning registration or marketing authorization

Fig. (4). Herbal medicine involvement of various legislative approaches.

3.1. The International Council for Harmonization

The Harmonization of traditional medicines listed in different pharmacopoeias such as Indian Pharmacopoeia, Chinese Pharmacopoeia, British Herbal Pharmacopoeia, and Ayurvedic Pharmacopoeia, *etc.* have the same specifications, that ensure safety, efficacy and quality of herbal medicines in different countries. The pharmacopoeia of China, Korea and Japan has listed similar herbal medicines, but under different specifications. The plant materials should have same families or species as per binomial nomenclature in every country [16]. India has about 8000 herbal companies, in which about the 5000 have Good

Manufacturing Practices (GMP) certified units and majority of them are medium or small-scale companies [17 - 19]. The drug regulatory agencies held an International conference in Madrid at 2004 and requested the regulatory agencies to work together to produce the product by sharing different National experience and information in herbal medicines [20, 21].

It has reported that about 4000 traditional medicines are used as remedies for treatment of human ailments based on evidence-based clinical practice. The European Commission have issued the directive 2004/24/EC for harmonizing the definition of traditional herbal medicinal products, by simplifying the registration procedure on herbal medicinal products [22 - 24]. However, the regulation of herbal products is an essential requirement in few countries which are isolated from jurisdiction of member countries and International agencies.

3.2. World Health Organization (WHO)

The drug-stability testing guidelines were published by the World Health Organization (WHO) in 1996 for pharmaceutical products [25 - 27]. WHO published different regulatory strategies in traditional medicine (TM) in 2002-2005 providing the framework to check traditional medicine and complementary alternative medicine (TM/CAM) for reducing morbidity and mortality in impoverished nation. The herbal medicine included in the International Conference on Drug Regulatory authorities (ICDRA) in fourth coherence in 1986-1989 for counter labelled of herbal products in health organization containing minimum basic guidelines in various legislation elements and its registration [28].

3.3. United States Food and Drug Administration (USFDA)

United States Food and Drug Administration (USFDA) along with ICH guidelines in 1998 comprehensively drafted the guideline for the herbal industry. According to the guidelines, stability testing of herbal drug substances and drug products requires stress testing which has to be tested under conditions as mentioned in the ICH guidelines. It has other recommendation for the Abbreviated New Drug Application (ANDAs) [29, 30]. The herbal medicines in the USA is less popular than major underdeveloped and the developing nation. The USFDA guidelines entitled for validation of chromatographic methods, methods of validation, analytical procedures, manufacturing, and chemistry and emphasize on stress testing. It also covers documentation for emphasized stress testing; use of samples in different medical scenarios [31 - 33].

3.4. European Medicines Agency (EMA)

The regulation system in traditional or herbal medicines, the Herbal Products Medicinal Committee (HPMC) constituted under the European Medicines Agency (EMA). HPMC is responsible for assessing and collating the data related to herbal substances and preparations. This also offers harmonization in the European market, introduced and simplified registration procedure for herbal medicinal products in European countries. HPMC is established under the Regulation (EC) No 726/2004 & Herbal Directive. It provides information about the use and safety conditions of herbal substances and their preparations. These regulations support harmonization of herbal products in the European market. The major roles of HPMC are the preparation of the monograph of herbal substance and preparation stating their safe conditions and therapeutic use; and preparation for the list of herbal substance, herbal preparation and herbal combinations that are marketed in European countries. HPMC consist of eight members and these are chairperson, members are appointed by the European state, Iceland and Norway and five co-opted members which provides other expertise [34].

4. REGULATORY GUIDELINES FOR HERBAL PRODUCTS

The first International appreciation of traditional medicinal products used in primary health care was well established in the Assertion of Alma-Ata. It means, inter alia, that "Primary health care relies, at local and referral levels, on health workers, including nurses, midwives, auxiliaries and communal workers as applicable, as well as traditional practitioners as needed". The safety issues emerged in the herbal medicinal product is due to largely unregulated growing market and a lack of effective quality assurance and control.

4.1. Guidelines for Regulated Market

The stringent lack under the guidance of efficacy assessment, quality assurance, quality control, safety monitoring and acquaintance on traditional medicine and alternative medicine (TM/CAM) are several aspects; that are found in the different regulatory systems. The resources finished in herbal medicinal products contain various phytochemical or other plant materials. The requirement for the registration and marketing authorization in herbal drugs regulated by marketing system such as EU, US, Singapore, Australia and Japan. In Europe, the Committee on Herbal Medicinal Products (HMPC) is the establishment in the European Medicines Agency (EMA) that simplified registration procedure for herbal medicinal products in EU member states under the regulation of herbal medicine directive 2004/24/EC (traditional herbal medicinal products directive) and regulation (EC) No 726/2004. In the United States, the FDA's The Center for Drug Evaluation and Research (CDER) categorized as the botanical drug definition in 201(g)(1)(B), Federal Food, Drug, and Cosmetic Act & different herbal product regulation, the Dietary Supplement Health and Education Act of 1994 (DSHEA) [35].

4.2. Guidelines for the Semi-regulated Market

For the semi-regulated countries follows their own regulatory and WHO under the guidelines for assessing quality of herbal medicines with reference to contaminants and residues at 2007. Many countries like India, China, South Africa, Saudi Arabia, Tanzania, South Korea, and Brazil are under semi regulatory market. Moreover, the countries like Singapore, Malaysia, Korea, Myanmar, Thailand, India, and China have their monographs for natural products. In India, herbal medicine manufactured as per guidance of Indian pharmacopoeia, Ayurvedic pharmacopoeia, Unani pharmacopoeia and Homoeopathic pharmacopoeia of India. The Indian system was separated for the essential medicines listed under traditional natural products in Ayurveda & Unani pharmacopoeias.

4.3. Guidelines for Non-regulatory Market

In the non-regulated market, every country follows the guidelines by WHO for herbal drug. Eighteen countries considered as the non-regulated market, which are mostly from African continent, and they have registration system for herbal medicine except Sri Lanka and Maldives. In Nepal and the Philippines, the monograph process has been started. The Philippines have the greater number of registered herbal drugs which is about 2500.

5. RECOMMENDATIONS ON HERBAL MEDICINE IN PHARMACOPOEIAS

5.1. United States Pharmacopoeia

In the United States, herbal natural medicines are not regulated as drugs, these products considered as the complementary/alternative medicines (CAM) or dietary supplements. The FDA constituted Dietary Supplement Health Education Act (DSHEA) in 1994 to support the regulations between the FDA and manufacturing products. However, the FDA has categorized CAM products into dietary supplements, food, food additives, new drug and new animal drug. The FDA's approved Centre for Botanical Drug Products *i.e.*, Drug Evaluation and Research (CDER) differentiates the botanical drugs as required for the New Drug Application (NDA) or could be marketed as Over-The-Counter (OTC) [35].

The USP Herbal Medicine Compendium (HMC) is an online compendium that ensures the quality of herbal ingredients used in the formulation. The HMC monographs on herbal drugs included specification for testing procedure and validated analytical procedure for the good quality assessment. USP now regulates the advancements in herbal ingredients through various standardization techniques as per HMC. The Herbal Medicine Compendium enclosed with 23 standard ingredients of herbal medicine except those from synthetic chemical, biotechnologically derived medicine and ingredients of animal origin. Now, HMC has made standard protocol readily available to the worldwide stakeholder which requires public standards for herbal medicinal ingredients. This standard protocol allows the stakeholder to keep a check on the low quality of the medicinal product (Fig. **5**).

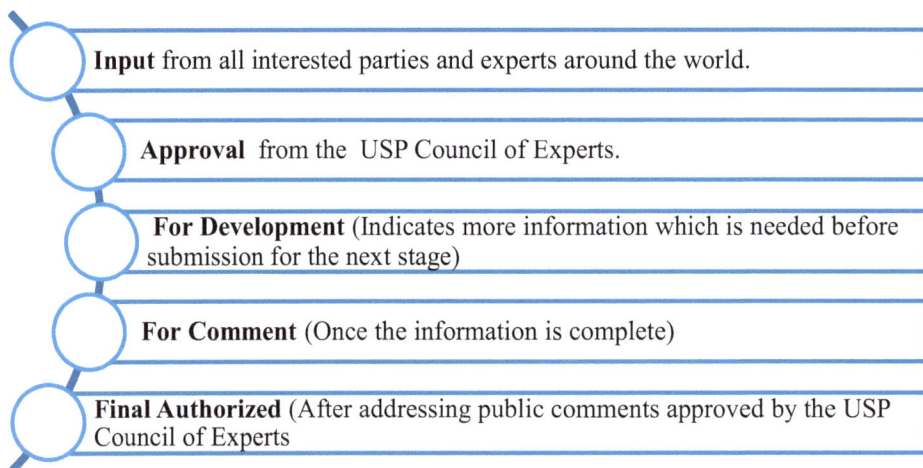

Input from all interested parties and experts around the world.

Approval from the USP Council of Experts.

For Development (Indicates more information which is needed before submission for the next stage)

For Comment (Once the information is complete)

Final Authorized (After addressing public comments approved by the USP Council of Experts

Fig. (5). Development of herbal medicine compendium.

5.2. Indian Pharmacopoeia

The Pharmacopoeia Commission for Indian Medicine and Homoeopathy (PCIM&H) was established in 2010 initially under Ministry in AYUSH, Government of the India. The main aim for the commission is to develop reference methods for the formulations that categorized as herbal medicine or traditional medicine in Ayurveda, Unani, Siddha and Homoeopathic systems. The

Indian Ayurvedic Pharmacopoeia Committee (APC) has published 45 monographs for drugs/formulation that are from plant origin. The latest edition of Ayurvedic Pharmacopoeia of India (API) has also included the standards for more than 550 single drugs and 152 other drug combinations (Table **2**).

Drug and Cosmetic (D&C) Act 1940 authorized API from 15.09.1964 to till now. Hence, all the monographs that are approved by APC and published in API, should comply with the quality guidelines described under D&C Act 1940. In 1978, first official Indian Ayurvedic Formulary was published in Ministry of the Health & Family Welfare, moreover 21 different drug formulations are included in 444 formulations are either in "Kasthaausadhis" (predominantly plant origin drugs) and "Rasaausadhi" (predominantly including metals and minerals). The Ayurvedic Pharmacopoeia of India was published in two parts: first part includes monographs of single drugs in different formulations and second part comprising monographs for fixed dosage forms or drug combination [36]. Apart from these pharmacopoeia's regulations, WHO have also published guidelines for quality control to be followed by herbal drug manufacturers. Various other regulations of the drug manufacturing and quality control described in different sections as mentioned in Table **3** [37].

Table 2. Ayurvedic Pharmacopoeia of India and their amendmen.

Ayurvedic Pharmacopoeia of India	Year of Publishing	Of Amendments
Part-I, volume-I	1989	80 monographs on single drugs of plant origin. Each monograph includes drug title along with its sources, occurrence, distribution and collection precautions, the water soluble or alcohol soluble. Extractives, specifications of lower limit have also been included
Part-I, volume-II	1999	Monograph on 78 drugs of plant origin following the same format
Part-I, volume-III	2003	In this volume total 100 monograph of plant origin drugs and also included advancement in thin layer chromatography(TLC), which is an identification test of the drug. TLC is included after identify; purity and strength in the monograph
Part-I, volume-IV	2004	Addition of 68 monograph of the plant origin drugs
Part-I, volume-V	2006	Encompass total 92 drugs of the plant origin in it
Part-I, volume-VI	2008	Include 101 new monographs out of which 97 are from plant origin and rest are of "Goghrita"(clarified cow's butter),"Guda" (jiggery)," Madhu" (honey) of the animal origin and "sarkara" (sugar)"jala(potable water)

(Table 2) cont.....

Part-I, volume-VII	2008	21 single mineral drugs, each monograph is prepared including drug names followed by its definition, synonyms, names in the other languages, board classification origin and occurrence, chemicals properties, physical properties
Part-I, volume-VIII	2011	This edition includes 60 new monographs out of which 15 are widely used single medicinal plant in different drugs as mentioned in Ayurveda. However, in the recent Rules 158(B) clause IV under the Drugs and cosmetics Act, 1940 provided the use of "Aushadhi Ghans", which includes wet and dry extracts of aqueous, hydro alcoholic origin along with other origins. The assay and chromatographic profile using Photochemical Reference Standards(PRS) have also been mentioned.
Part-I-volume-IX	2016	Includes 45 monographs for drugs of plant origin, the preparation and standardization of crude extract drugs and drugs with hydro alcoholic and aqueous extracts with their chromatographic fingerprint
Part-II-volume-I	2007	50 new monographs drug formulated in combined mixture
Part-II-volume-II	2008	Inclusion of 51 monographs
Part-II-volume-III	2010	51 monographs for drugs formulated in the combined mixture
TLC Atlas of Pharmacopoeial drugs Part-I, Volume-I	2009	80 new monographs
Microscopy and macroscopy Atlas of Pharmacopoeial drugs Part-I, Volume-I	2011	80 monographs
Microscopy and macroscopy Atlas of Pharmacopoeial drugs Part-I, Volume-V	2009	92 monographs

Table 3. WHO guidelines for quality control of herbal drugs.

Section	Regulation
Sec.33-C	Ayurvedic, Siddha, and Unani Drugs Technical Advisory Board
Sec.33-D	The Ayurvedic, Siddha, and Unani Drugs Consultative Committee
Sec.33-E	If Ayurvedic, Siddha, and Unani drug deemed to Be misbranded
Sec.33-3F	If Ayurvedic, Siddha, and Unani drug deemed to be adulterated
Sec.33-EEA	If Ayurvedic, Siddha, and Unani drug deemed to be spurious
Section-33-EEB	Regulation of Manufacture for Sale of Ayurvedic, Siddha, and Unani (ASU) Drugs
Section-33-EEC	Prohibition of Manufacture and Sale of Certain Ayurvedic, Siddha, And Unani Drugs

(Table 3) cont.....

Section-33-EED	Power of Central Government to Prohibit Manufacture *etc.*, of Ayurvedic, Siddha, and Unani Drugs in Public Interest
Form24-D	Licensing Authorities
Form24-E	Loan License

The state licensing authorities of Ayurvedic, Siddha and Unani (ASU) drugs assures the compliance by all ASU drug manufacturers in accordance to provisions of Rule 161(1) and 161(2) *i.e.* related to the true listed for the all ingredients. In ASU formulation under provision of Rule 169 and 127 permits the use excipients and color, respectively. As on April 1, 2010 Government of India had made mandatory to mention the expiry date of Ayurvedic formulation [38].

5.3. Chinese Pharmacopoeia

In China, Natural medicinal products marketed and manufactured in accordance with Chinese Pharmacopoeia (ChP) and other FD Approved specifications. In China, the herbal products can be registered as functional drugs or food under Governance for the State Food & Drug Administration (SFDA). Chinese Medicine Ordinance (chapter 549 of the laws of Hong Kong) has specified 31 types of potent or toxic Chinese Herbal Medicines (CHM) in Schedule 1. The CHM has been classified in four main categories, such as western medicine, food, proprietary Chinese medicines and consumer goods. CHM should comply (foods and drugs) for the Public Health and Municipal Services Ordinance (chapter 132 of the laws of Hong Kong) [39]. The Government of China and Ministry of health play an important role in healthcare system in Chinese population. Chinese Pharmacopoeia (ChP) has monographs for the standardization of drugs and the general requirements of testing methods. After the compilation of pharmacopoeia, it is approved by China Food Drug Administration (CFDA). First Chinese Pharmacopoeia was published in 1952 by Ministry of Health. Different editions of Chinese Pharmacopoeia along with the amendments illustrated in Table **4**. People's Republic of China enacted the law in 2001 that governs the "State Drug Administration" (SDA), which provides medicinal products with good quality, efficacy and safety. It is mandatory for the manufacturer to comply with the guidelines legislated by SDA. The DNA bar-coding system is generating various reliable techniques for herbal authentication. In China, DNA bar-coding system *i.e.* BOMMD (Bar-code of Medicinal Materials Database) integrate TCM taxonomy and pharmacological properties, because web DNA barcode *i.e.* Medicinal Materials DNA Barcode Database (MMDBD) integrates medical parts, herbal resources and adulterant information. MMDBD holds over 1,600 species of medicinal materials listed in the American Herbal Pharmacopoeia and Chinese Pharmacopoeia up to May 2014 [40, 41].

Table 4. Herbal monographs and amendments of Chinese Pharmacopoeia.

Pharmacopoeia Edition	Publishing Year	Amendments in Herbal Drugs
2nd	1963	446 monographs of Chinese medicaments and 197 monographs of patent preparation
3rd	1977	882 and 270 monographs of Chinese herbal medicine and Chinese traditional patent preparation respectively
4th	1985	506 monographs of Chinese medicament and 207 monographs of Chinese patent preparation
5th	1990	509 monographs of Chinese medicament and 275 monographs of Chinese patent preparation
6th	1995	522 monographs of Chinese traditional crude drug, 398 monographs of Chinese patent preparation
7th	2000	-
8th	-	-
9th	2010	1386 new monographs and 2237 revised monographs
10th	2015	440 new monographs, 517 revision and 7 rejection in volume-I, 492 new monographs, 415 revision and 28 rejection in volume-II and 13 new monographs and 105 revision.

5.4. European Union Pharmacopoeia

In Europe, a Committee for Herbal Medicinal Product (HMPC) established for the European Medicines Agency in London in 2004 in September month. This Committee was established to harmonize the manufacture & trade for the traditional herbal medicines in the European market. The HMPC committed to issue or publish the monographs and guidelines related to herbal medicinal products. The HMPC comprises 33 members out of which 28 members represent European Union and one each from Norway & Iceland (EEA-EFTA states). Remaining five members of HMPC represent different domains of science. The HMP functions in collaboration with European Directorate for the Quality of Medicines and Health Care (EDQM) and various scientific authorities in Europe and around the world. The scientific experts of European Commission, EU candidates (Albania, Bosnia, FYROM, Herzegovina, Kosovo, Montenegro, Serbia and Turkey) and EDQM (European Directorate for the Quality of Medicines and Health Care) take part in different meetings of HMPS as official observers [42]. On 26th April, 2007 the French regulation (Ordinance no. 2007613) implemented the Directive 2004/24 which demonstrated that the HMPC was mainly responsible for the evaluation, registration & authorization for the herbal products. The French Directive 2004/24 further amended for the legislation in Directive

2001/83/EC, that allows the marketing of various medicinal products only after regulatory parameters concerned with quality, safety and efficacy [43, 44].

CONCLUSION

Herbal products are generally used for skin care, healthcare and as a dietary supplement. Across the globe, pharmaceutical industries are emphasizing on research related to herbal products due to economic reasons. Before marketing, manufacturing system should have information about the regulatory framework laid down by other countries. Challenges faced by regulatory bodies are towards the improvement of maximum safety, quality and efficacy of various herbal drugs. In recent years, regulation towards herbal medicine is much more concerned about safety and quality; many guidelines have been published and amended for the same. Different regulatory agencies have different guidelines for the potentially active ingredient. Harmonization of regulatory guidance of various agencies will ensure the uniformity in standards in herbal medical products in the pharmaceutical industry world-wide and it will enhance the herbal product trade within countries.

ABBREVIATIONS

API	Ayurvedic Pharmacopoeia of India
BHP	British Herbal Pharmacopoeia
CAM	Complementary Alternative Medicine
GMP	Good Manufacturing Practice
FDA	Food and Drug Administration
IP	Indian Pharmacopoeia
TIM	Traditional Indian Medicine
TKM	Traditional Korean Medicine
TCM	Traditional Chinese Medicine
TJM	Traditional Japanese Medicine
UMS	Unani Medical System
WHO	World Health Organization

CONSENT FOR PUBLICATION

Not applicable.

CONFLICT OF INTEREST

The author(s) confirms that there is no conflict of interest.

ACKNOWLEDGEMENTS

Declared none.

REFERENCES

[1]   Mankar SD, Gholap VD, Zenda TP, Dighe RS. Drug regulatory agencies in India, USA, Europe and Japan-a Review. Inter J Inst Pharm Sci 2014; 4(2): 288-97.

[2]   Lahlou M. Screening of natural products for drug discovery. Expert Opin Drug Discov 2007; 2(5): 697-705.
[http://dx.doi.org/10.1517/17460441.2.5.697] [PMID: 23488959]

[3]   Newman DJ, Cragg GM. Natural products as sources of new drugs from 1981 to 2014. J Nat Prod 2016; 79(3): 629-61.
[http://dx.doi.org/10.1021/acs.jnatprod.5b01055] [PMID: 26852623]

[4]   Bate R, Tren R, Mooney L, *et al.* Pilot study of essential drug quality in two major cities in India. PLoS One 2009; 4(6)e6003
[http://dx.doi.org/10.1371/journal.pone.0006003] [PMID: 19547757]

[5]   Imran M, Abul K, Mohammad F. Rashid, Tabrez S, Mushtaq A Shah. Clinical research regulation in India-history, development, initiatives, challenges and controversies: still long way to go. J Pharm Biol Sci 2013; 5: 1.

[6]   Philip S, Ansa P. The scope of regulatory affairs in the pharmaceutical industry, Hygeia. J Med 2010; 2(1): 1-6.

[7]   Budhwar V, Yadav S, Manjusha CH. Nitesh. A Comprehension study on regulation of herbal drug in USA, European Union and India. Inter J Drug Reg Affairs 2017; 5(4): 8-17.
[http://dx.doi.org/10.22270/ijdra.v5i4.205]

[8]   Quality control methods for medicinal plant material. Geneva: World Health Organization 1998; pp. 8-78.

[9]   Verma N. Herbal Medicines: Regulation and practice in Europe, United States and India. Int J Heb Med 2013; 1(4): 1-5.

[10]   Shivam L, Amol K, Mayur G, Shreyas D. Cooperation Scheme (PIC/S) to promote a globally accepted GMP. Role of drug regulatory affairs in Pharma industry. W J Pharm Res 2015; 6(6): 615-25.

[11]   Health Canada. Natural health products regulations. https://www.canada.ca/en/health-canada/services/ drugs-health-products/natural-non-prescription.html.

[12]   Health Canada. Pathway for Licensing Natural health products making modern Health Claims. https://www.canada.ca/content/dam/hc-sc/migration/hc-sc/dhp-mps/alt_formats/pdf/prodnatur/ legislation/docs/modern-eng.pdf.

[13]   Farrell J, Ries NM, Boon H. Pharmacists and Natural Health Products: A systematic analysis of professional responsibilities in Canada. Pharm Pract (Granada) 2008; 6(1): 33-42.
[http://dx.doi.org/10.4321/S1886-36552008000100006] [PMID: 22282720]

[14]   Anis AH. Pharmaceutical policies in Canada: another example of federal-provincial discord. CMAJ 2000; 162(4): 523-6.
[PMID: 10701389]

[15]   MacLeod-Glover N. An explanatory policy analysis of legislative change permitting pharmacists in Alberta, Canada, to prescribe. Int J Pharm Pract 2011; 19(1): 70-8.
[http://dx.doi.org/10.1111/j.2042-7174.2010.00074.x] [PMID: 21235661]

[16]   Jayasuriya DC. The regulation of medicinal plants a preliminary review of the selected aspects of national legislation.

[17] De Smet PAGM. Should herbal medicine-like products be licensed as medicines. BMJ 1995; 310(6986): 1023-4.
[http://dx.doi.org/10.1136/bmj.310.6986.1023] [PMID: 7728046]

[18] Choi DW, Kim JH, Cho SY, Kim DH, Chang SY. Regulation and quality control of herbal drugs in Korea. Toxicology 2002; 181-182: 581-6.
[http://dx.doi.org/10.1016/S0300-483X(02)00487-0] [PMID: 12505370]

[19] Working group on "Access to health system including AYUSH", Eleventh five-year plan (2007-2012) Government of India planning commission. https://niti.gov.in/planningcommission.gov.in/docs/ aboutus/committee/wrkgrp11/wg11_hayush.pdf.

[20] WHO. World Health Organization international standard terminologies on traditional medicine in the western pacific region, 2007. https://apps.who.int/iris/bitstream/handle/10665/206952/97892 90612487_eng.pdf?sequence=1&isAllowed=y.

[21] Department of AYUSH, ministry of health and family welfare, Government of India. www.indianmedicine.nic.in

[22] World Health Organization. National policy on 11. World Health Organization. 2005; 11: pp. 5-6.

[23] Uppsala Monitoring Centre. Herbal drug side reaction, 2009. https://www.who-umc.org/.

[24] Association of the European self-medication industry (AESGP) Legal and regulatory framework European Self-medication industry (AESGP). 2010; 7.

[25] ICH, Q1A (R2) stability testing of new drug substances and products. Geneva. Switzerland. 2003. https://www.ema.europa.eu/en/documents/scientific-guideline/ich-q-1-r2-stability-testing-new-drug-substances-products-step-5_en.pdf.

[26] World Health Organization. WHO traditional strategy, 2002-2005 Document WHO/EDM/TRM/2002 1 Geneva World Health Organization. 2002.

[27] WHO, Expert committee on specification for pharmaceutical preparations, WHO technical report series, No. 863, thirty fourth reports, annex5-guidelines for stability testing of pharmaceutical products containing well established drug substances in conventional dosages form. Geneva, Switzerland, 1996. https://www.paho.org/hq/dmdocuments/2008/6_Annex_5_report_34.pdf.

[28] WHO, Expert committee on specification for pharmaceutical preparation, WHO technical report series 969, Annex 5, guidelines for registration of fixed-dose combination medicinal products, appendix3, pharmaceutical development (or preformulation) studies, Geneva, Switzerland, 2009.

[29] WHO. Guidelines on submission of documentation for a multisource (Generic) finished pharmaceutical product (FPP): Quality part (Draft for comments), Geneva, Switzerland, 2013. https://www.who.int/medicines/areas/quality_safety/quality_assurance/Quality-QAS1- -522Rev1_09072013.pdf.

[30] EMA, CHMP. Guidelines on stability testing for application for variation to a marketing authorization, London, UK, 2012. https://www.ema.europa.eu/en/documents/scientific-guideline/guideline-stabili-y-testing-applications-variations-marketing-authorisation-revision-2_en.pdf.

[31] USFDA, Guidance for industry: stability testing of drug substances and drug products. Rockville's, 1998.

[32] Kuipers SE, Farnsworth NR, Fong HMS, Segelman AB, Herbal medicines-A continuing world trend presentation at the 1st world federation of proprietary medicine manufacturing Asia Pacific Regional meeting, Jakarta. http://digicollection.org/hss/fr/d/Jwhozip57e/6.html.

[33] USFDA. Guidance for industry: analytical procedures and methods validation; chemistry manufacturing and control documentation, Rockville, USA, 2000. https://www.fda.gov/files/drugs/ published/Analytical-Procedures-and-Methods-Validation-for-Drugs-and-Biologics.pdf.

[34] USFADA. Centre for drug evaluation and research (CDER). Reviewer guidance: validation of

chromatographic methods, Rockville, USA, 1994. https://www.fda.gov/regulatory-information/searc-
-fda-guidance-documents/reviewer-guidance-validation-chromatographic-methods.

[35]   Reflection paper on stability testing of herbal medicinal products and traditional herbal medicinal
        products (Ref. EMA/HMPC/3626), 2009

[36]   Joshi VK, Joshi A, Dhiman KS. The Ayurvedic Pharmacopoeia of India, development and
        perspectives. J Ethnopharmacol 2017; 197: 32-8.
        [http://dx.doi.org/10.1016/j.jep.2016.07.030] [PMID: 27404231]

[37]   Mukherjee PK. Exploring Botanicals in Indian System of Medicine-Regulatory Perspectives. Clinical
        Research and Regulatory Affairs. 2003; 20(3): 249-64.
        [http://dx.doi.org/10.1081/CRP-120023840]

[38]   Mondal S. Quality, Safety, and Efficacy of herbal products through regulatory harmonization. Drug
        Inf J 2011; 45: 45-53.
        [http://dx.doi.org/10.1177/009286151104500105]

[39]   Xiaoqing F, Salmon JW. Herbal Medicine Regulation in China, Germany, and the United States.
        Integr Med (Encinitas) 2010; 5.

[40]   Chau CF, Wu SH. The development of regulations of Chinese herbal medicines for both medicinal and
        food uses. Trends Food Sci Technol 2006; 17: 313-23.
        [http://dx.doi.org/10.1016/j.tifs.2005.12.005]

[41]   Liu SH, Chuang WC, Lam W, Jiang Z, Cheng YC. Safety surveillance of traditional Chinese
        medicine: current and future. Drug Saf 2015; 38(2): 117-28.
        [http://dx.doi.org/10.1007/s40264-014-0250-z] [PMID: 25647717]

[42]   Ioanna C, Werner K, Gioacchino C. Regulation of herbal medicinal products in the EU: an up-to-date
        scientific review. Phytochem Rev 2014.

[43]   Verma N. Herbal Medicines: Regulation and Practice in Europe, United States and India. Int J Herbal
        Med 2013; 1(4): 1-5.

[44]   Benzi G, Ceci A. Herbal medicines in European regulation. Pharmacol Res 1997; 35(5): 355-62.
        [http://dx.doi.org/10.1006/phrs.1997.0132] [PMID: 9299199]

CHAPTER 10

Phytochemicals for the Treatment of Human Diseases

Javed Ahamad[1,*], Subasini Uthirapathy[2], Kamran Javed Naquvi[3], Muath Sh. Mohammed Ameen[4], Esra T. Anwer[4], Abdul Samad[5] and Mohammad Shabib Akhtar[6]

[1] *Department of Pharmacognosy, Faculty of Pharmacy, Tishk International University, Erbil, Kurdistan Region, Iraq*

[2] *Department of Pharmacology, Faculty of Pharmacy, Tishk International University, Kurdistan Region, Iraq*

[3] *Department of Pharmacognosy & Phytochemistry, Faculty of Pharmaceutical Sciences, Rama University, Rama City, Mandhana, Kanpur (Uttar Pradesh) - 209 217, India*

[4] *Department of Pharmaceutics, Faculty of Pharmacy, Tishk International University, KRG, Iraq*

[5] *Department of Pharmaceutical Chemistry, Faculty of Pharmacy, Tishk International University, KRG, Iraq*

[6] *Department of Clinical Pharmacy, College of Pharmacy, Najran University, Kingdom of Saudi Arabia*

Abstract: Medicinal plants are a major source of remedies for the treatment of human ailments in under-developed and developing countries. Traditional or alternative medicines were practiced in ancient civilizations for the cure of human ailments. In recent years, natural products play a vital role in drug discovery for life-threatening ailments like cancer, malaria, diabetes, and cardiovascular problems. Due to the advancement of scientific techniques, isolated phytochemicals can be developed as a medicine for lifestyle and chronic disorders. Herbal medicinal products are also developed for effective treatment of several diseases like cancer, malaria, diabetes, cardiovascular complications, *etc*. Recently,drug discovery from plants for the treatment of cancer has become more focused, leading to the discovery of novel anticancer drugs such as paclitaxel, docetaxel, topotecan, irinotecan, vincristine, and vinblastine, *etc*. In this book chapter, we have discussed important medicinal plants and bioactive natural products for the treatment or management of diabetes mellitus, cancer, obesity, and cardiovascular complications.

Keywords: Bioactive Phytochemicals, Cancer, Cardiovascular Complications, Drug Discovery, Diabetes Mellitus, Herbal Medicine, Natural Product.

* **Corresponding author Javed Ahamad:** Department of Pharmacognosy, Faculty of Pharmacy, Tishk International University, Erbil, Kurdistan Region, Iraq; E-mails: jas.hamdard@gmail.com; javed.ahamad@tiu.edu.iq

1. INTRODUCTION

Higher plants fulfill the significant human requirements such as food, shelter, clothes, and remedies for the cure of ailments [1]. Ethnobotany and ethnopharmacology utilize plants for the treatment of various ailments based upon the long history of their use by humans. Natural products derived from medicinal plants considered safe and effective compared to modern synthetic drugs. Because these natural resources are distributed throughout the world and grown in crop fields, they are comparatively cheap to synthetic drugs. The WHO estimates about traditional medicines states that approximately 80% of developing and developed countries rely on herbal or traditional medicine for their primary health care needs [2, 3].The plant has advantages in drug discovery based on along history of use by humans as food and medicine. So ,the drugs discovered from medicinal plants are supposed to have fewer side effects compared to modern drugs. In recent years,the discovery of several novel and potent anticancer (*e.g.* taxols, vincristine, vinblastine, camptothecin *etc.*), antimalarials (*e.g.* artemisinins, quinine *etc.*), antihypertensive (*e.g.* reserpine), cardiotonics (*e.g.* digoxin) *etc* realizes the importance of natural resources as the major source of drug discovery [3]. Hence, public, academic, and government interest is increasing nowadays in traditional medicine [4]. Alternative or traditional medicines use plants and have become a significant source for the treatment of chronic diseases and disorders of humans [5]. Current therapy to alleviate cancer and metabolic disorders such as diabetes mellitus, cardiovascular complications is not optimal, and thus, efforts have been made to develop effective and better drugs from natural sources [6, 7]. Isolated bioactive phytochemicals and their derivatives also approved for the treatment of human ailments' such as malaria, cancer, diabetes, *etc.* (Table **1**). In this book chapter, we discussed separately natural products used in the treatment of diabetes mellitus, cancer, cardiovascular complications, obesity, and natural products with anti-inflammatory and antioxidant activities.

2. HERBAL MEDICINES WITH ANTIDIABETIC ACTIVITY

Diabetes mellitus (DM) is a chronic metabolic disorder, associated with obesity and cardiovascular complications, which emerged as the major killer for mankind [8]. Sedentary lifestyle and obesity nowadays have become a major factor in the development of type 2 DM, and diabetes is the primary cause of other severe health problems such as diabetic retinopathy, neuropathy and cardiovascular complications such as atherosclerosis, stroke, peripheral vascular diseases, coronary artery diseases and these lead to angina and diabetic myonecrosis [9]. In recent years, it has been observed that the number of DM patients worldwide increased significantly. Current therapies for the treatment of type 2 DM and related cardiovascular complications are not optimal and having more adverse effects, and thus efforts should be made to develop effective and safe drugs from natural sources. In recent years, the use of traditional medicines in the modern way has expanded globally, and it's gaining popularity day by day. Medicinal plants have been widely used for therapeutic purposes due to the expensive and unaffordability of modern medicines in the rural areas of developing and undeveloped countries compared to herbal remedies, which are cheap and considered as safe [10 - 12]. In pursuit of new medications for diabetes mellitus treatment and associated complications, several researchers emphasize the utilization of natural products and their secondary metabolites. Ethnobotanical knowledge reports about 800 plants that possess the antidiabetic potential [13].

Table 1. Natural products (N) and natural products derivative (ND) approved by US-FDA for the treatment of human diseases [7].

Clinical Class	Natural Products/ Natural Product Derivatives	Year of Approval
Antibacterial drugs	Carumonam (N)	1988
	Daptomycin (N)	2003
	Fidaxomicin (N)	2011
	Fosfomycin trometamol (N)	1988
	Isepamicin (N)	1988
	Micronomicin sulphate (N)	1982
	Miokamycin (N)	1985
	Mupirocin (N)	1985
	Netilimicin sulphate (N)	1981
	RV-11(N)	1989
	Teicoplanin (N)	1988
Antiparasitic drugs	Artemisinin (N)	1987
	Arteether (ND)	2000
	Artemether (ND)	1987
	Artesunate (ND)	1987
	Mefloquine HCI (ND)	1985

(Table 1) cont.....

Clinical Class	Natural Products/ Natural Product Derivatives	Year of Approval
Anticancer drugs	Paclitaxel (N)	1993
	Docetaxel (ND)	1995
	Solamargines (NB)	1989
	Belotecan hydrochloride (ND)	2004
	Cabazitaxel (ND)	2010
	Etoposide (ND)	1980
	Etoposide phosphate (ND)	1996
	Irinotecan hydrochloride (ND)	1994
	Topotecan HCl (ND)	1996
	Vinblastine (N)	1967
	Vincristine (N)	1963
	Vindesine (ND)	1979
	Vinorelbine (ND)	1989
	Vinflunine (ND)	2010
Antidiabetic drugs	Voglibose (N)	1994
	Acarbose (ND)	1990
	Miglitol (ND)	1998
Antiviral drugs	Oseltamivir (ND)	1999
	Zanamivir (ND)	1999
	Enfuvirtide (ND)	2003
	Laninamivir octanoate (ND)	2010
Antifungal drugs	Anidulafungin (ND)	2006
	Caspofungin acetate (ND)	2001
	Micafungin sodium (ND)	2002

2.1. Current Therapies for Diabetes Mellitus

Newman and Cragg, reported that a total of 52 drug molecules was discovered from 1981 to 2014 and out of which 7 drugs are natural product or natural product derivatives; 23 from the biological origin and 4 drugs from the synthetic origin. Eleven drugs were synthesized that mimic natural products, and 7 drugs were indeed synthesized from natural products as a pharmacophore for the treatment of diabetes mellitus [7]. Type 1 and 2 DM are incurable chronic conditions but have been treatable since insulin became medically available in 1921. Type 1 DM mainly treated by the administration of exogenous insulin and exercise. Type 2 DM was treated by oral hypoglycemics and insulin supplementation. For improvement of insulin availability, mostly exogenous insulin preparations, sulphonylureas, and meglitinides are used. For the treatment of insulin resistance, mostly biguanides, thiazolidinediones, dipeptidyl peptidase IV inhibitors (DPP-IV), and sodium-dependent glucose transporter inhibitors (SGLTi,s) are used.

2.2. Bioactive Phytochemicals with Antidiabetic Activity

2.2.1. Charantin

Charantin (mixture of β-sitosterol glucoside and 5,25-stigmastadienol glucoside) is obtained from the fruits of *Momordica charantia* Linn. (Cucurbitaceae) and commonly known as bitter gourd and karela. In India, its fruit juice is considered a magical remedy for the treatment of diabetes mellitus [14]. Several herbal formulations marketed in India predominantly contain its extract. Bitter gourd contains cucurbitane type triterpenoids in which charantin Fig. (**1**) is the major one responsible for antidiabetic effect. Several researchers confirm its antidiabetic activity in animal and clinical models [17 - 20].

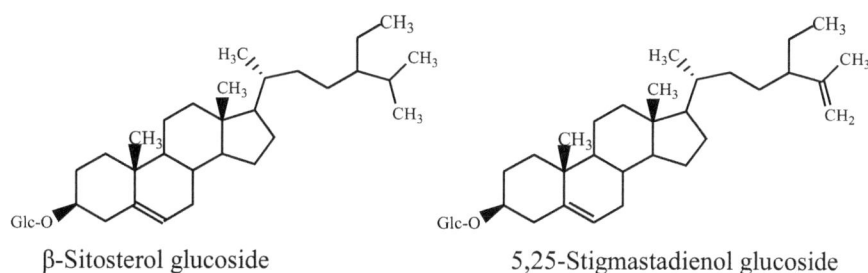

β-Sitosterol glucoside   5,25-Stigmastadienol glucoside

Fig. (1). Chemical structure of Charantin (a mixture of β-sitosterol glucoside and 5,25-stigmastadienol glucoside).

2.2.2. Swertiamarin

Swertiamarin is obtained from *Enicostemma littorale* Linn. (Gentianaceae). *E. littorale* is common ingredient of several Ayurvedic medicines for the treatment of diabetes. *E. littorale* contains swertiamarin (Fig. **2**), a secoiridoid glycoside as the major chemical constituent. The role of *E. littorale* and swertiamarin in the treatment of diabetes and hyperlipidemia was reported by several researchers. The authors also determined beneficial effects of swertiamarin and erythrocentaurin (swertiamarin metabolites), against post-prandial hyperglycemia in the *in-vitro* and *in-vivo* antidiabetic models [5, 21]. The antidiabetic and antihyperlipidemic effects of swertiamarin were also established by several researchers in animal models [22, 23].

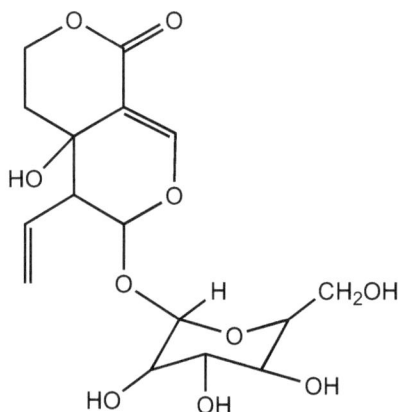

Fig. (2). Chemical structure of Swertiamarin.

2.2.3. Gymnemic Acids

It is a mixture of about 12 gymnemic acids that are isolated from *Gymnema sylvestre* R.Br. (Asclepiadaceae) and commonly known as Gurmar. In India, it is traditionally used for the cure of diabetes. Gurmar contains pentacyclic triterpenic glycosides known as gymnemic acids (Fig. **3**). Different arylated gymnemic acids were isolated and evaluated against carbohydrate metabolizing enzymes in *in-vitro* studies, and the study results supported traditional claim as these gymnemic acid derivatives were found potent inhibitors of carbohydrate metabolizing enzymes [24, 25]. Several other researchers determined the beneficial effects of gymnemic acids and their derivatives in the treatment of diabetes in various animal models [26, 27].

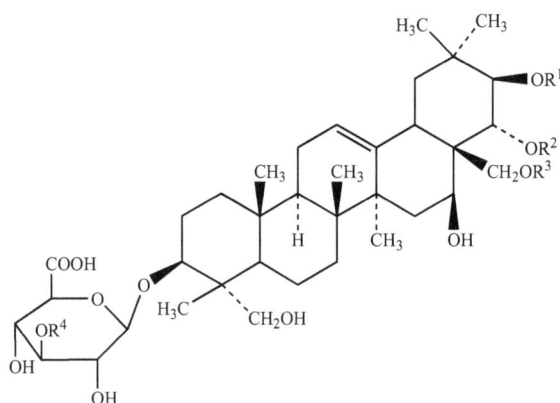

Fig. (3). Chemical structures of different types of Gymnemic acids.

Gymnemic Acids	R¹	R²	R³	R⁴
I	-tga	-H	-Ac	-H
II	-mba	-H	-Ac	-H
III	-mba	-H	-H	-H
IV	-tga	-H	-H	-H
V	-tga	-tga	-H	-H
VIII	-mba	-H	-H	-OG
IX	-tga	-H	-H	-OG
X	-H	-H	-Ac	-H
XI	-tga	-H	-tga	-H
XII	-tga	-H	-Ac	-glu
XIII	-H	-H	-mba	-H
XIV	-H	-H	-tga	-H

(where: -Ac = acetyl; -Glu = glucose; -OG = β-arabino-2-hexulopyranosyl, tga = tigloyl, mba = 2-methyl butyroyl)

2.2.4. Oleuropein

Oleuropeinis isolated from Olive (*Olea europaea* Linn., Oleaceae), which predominantly grows in Mediterranean countries. Olives are considered as important part of diet in Arabian countries. The olive tree is a globally prevalent plant specie and has been described as one of the most important cultivated crops [1]. Oleuropein Fig. (**4**) is a predominant phenolic compound present in Olive leaves, which is responsible for its beneficial antidiabetic activity [28]. Several researchers proved its beneficial effects in diabetes mellitus in preclinical and clinical studies [29 - 33].

2.2.5. Berberine

Berberine is isolated from stem and root barks of *Berberis* species (Berberidaceae), which is commonly known as *Daruhaldi*. In the Indian subcontinent, Berberis is used for the treatment of diabetes and liver complications. Ahamad *et al.*, reported its beneficial antidiabetic effects in animal models [34]. *B. aristata* has exhibited a significant antidiabetic activity in the glucose tolerance test [35]. Berberine Fig. (**5**), an isoquinoline alkaloid found in *Berberis* spp. promotes glucose consumption. In the *in-vitro* study berberine and metformin in combination enhanced glucose metabolism by stimulating glycolysis and AMPK activation [36].

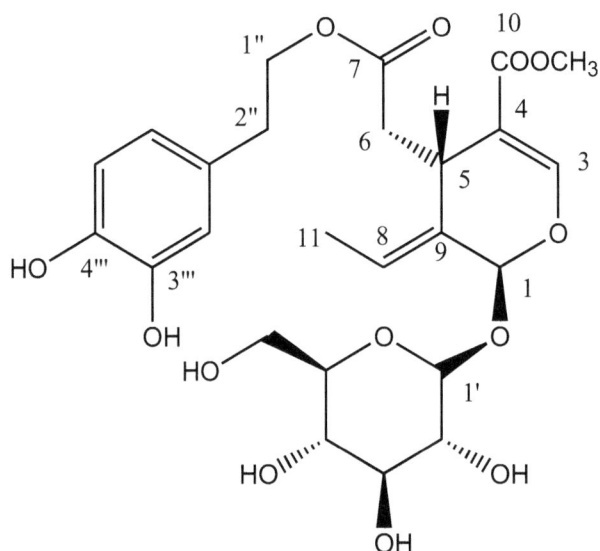

Fig. (4). Chemical structure of Oleuropein.

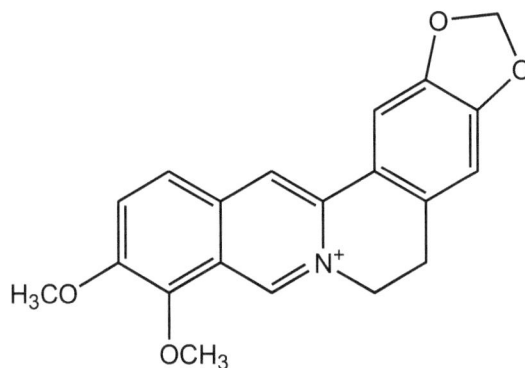

Fig. (5). Chemical structure of Berberine.

2.2.6. 4-Hydroxyisoleucine

It is obtained from the seeds of *Trigonella foenum-graecum* Linn. (Papilionaceae, commonly known as Fenugreek). In the Indian subcontinent, traditionally Fenugreek is used as a spice and cultivated throughout the sub-country [37, 38]. Fenugreek has been reported as a potent antidiabetic and hypocholesterolemic agent [39]. 4-Hydroxyisoleucine Fig. (**6**) and trigonelline are major chemical constituents responsible for its antidiabetic effects [40, 41].

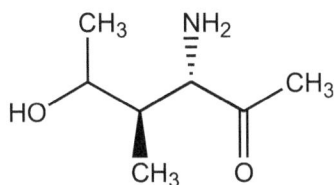

Fig. (6). Chemical structure of 4-Hydroxyisoleucine.

2.2.7. Epicatechin

It is isolated from the barks of *Pterocarpus marsupium* Roxb. (Leguminosae). Since ancient times *Pterocarpus* has been traditionally used for the treatment of diabetes in the Indian subcontinent [42]. Epicatechin Fig. (7) is considered as primary chemical compound responsible for its anti-diabetic effect. Preclinical studies in animal models proved it,s efficacy in diabetes [43].

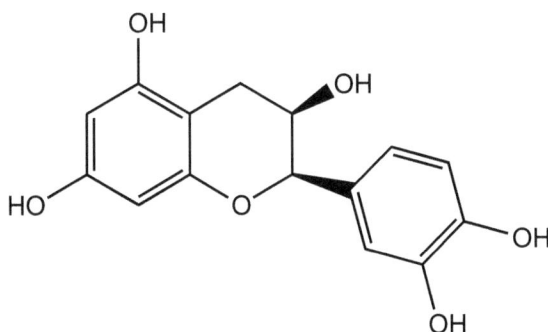

Fig. (7). Chemical structure of Epicatechin.

2.2.8. β-Sitosterol

β-Sitosterol and several flavonoids such a squercetin, kaempferol, myricetin, gallic acid, and ellagic acid have been isolated from *Eugenia jambolana* Linn. (Myrtaceae) which is popularly known as Jamun or Indian blackberry and has been indicated in Ayurveda. It is very well known for its antidiabetic effects. In accordance with its reputation as antidiabetic plant in traditional medicine, *E. jambolana* has been reported in both experimental animal models and clinical studies [44]. In Table **2**, natural products with antidiabetic activity are summarized.

Table 2. Bioactive phytochemicals with antidiabetic activity.

Phytochemicals	Source	Pharmacological Action	References
S-allyl cysteine	*Allium sativum*	Antidiabetic	[45]
Peptides and charantin	*Momordica charantia*	It has insulin secretagogue and insulinomimetic activities. Decreases insulin resistance Inhibits α-amylase and α-glucosidase enzyme	[19, 46, 47]
Swertiamarin	*Enicostemma littorale*	It increases insulin secretion. Increases the activity of hexokinase. Antihyperlipidaemic activity. Inhibits α-amylase and α-glucosidase enzyme	[5, 48]
Gymnemic acids and derivatives	*Gymnema sylvestre*	It increases insulin secretion. It repairs and regenerates β-cells of pancreas. Inhibits α-glucosidase enzyme	[24, 25, 49, 50]
Oleuropein	*Olea europaea*	Decrease fasting blood glucose levels. Increases insulin secretion and sensitivity	[30, 51]
Berberine	*Berberis aristata*	Increases glycolysis	[36]
4-hydroxy-isoleucine	*Trigonella foenum graecum*	Increases insulin release	[40]
Epicatechin	*P. marsupium*	Insulinomimetic	[43]
Resveratrol	*Veratrum grandiflorum, Polygonum cuspidatum*	Increases insulin secretion and sensitivity. Increases glucose metabolism	[52]
Betavulgarosides	*Beta vulgaris*	Hypoglycaemic	[41]
Quercetin	-	Prevents and protect β-cells of pancreas	[53]
Genistein	*Genista tinctoria*	Increases insulin secretion	[54, 55]
Methyl caffeate	*Solanum torvum*	Antihyperglycemic activity and antidiabetic effect	[56]
Macatannins A and B	*Macaranga tanarius*	Inhibits α-glucosidase enzyme	[57]

Phytochemicals	Source	Pharmacological Action	References
Cyanidin 3-glucoside	*Myrica rubra*	Inhibits insulin resistance	[58]
Chebulinic acid derivatives	*Capparis moonii*	Insulinomimetic activity	[59]
Kaempferol	-	Protects β-cells oxidative damage	[60]
Salacinol and Kotalanol	*Salaciareticulata, S. oblonga, S. chinensis*	Inhibits α-glucosidase enzyme	[61]
Methylswertianin and bellidifolin	*Swertia punicea*	Antidiabetic effect	[62]

3. HERBAL MEDICINES WITH ANTICANCER ACTIVITY

Drug discovery's paradigm has shifted significantly in recent years towards research exploring the drugs with antitumor and cytotoxic activity. From 1981 to 2014, total 174 drug molecules were approved, out of which 53% were only obtained from either directly from natural products or derived from natural resources [13]. Natural products lead to the discovery of several vital anticancer drugs, such as paclitaxel, docetaxel, etoposide, irinotecan, *etc*. In recent years, cancer became a leading cause of human death worldwide. National Cancer Institute estimated new cases of cancer 1,762,450 and 606,880 deaths for 2019 [63]. Cancer causes significant economic and social burdens to almost every country in the world. The major treatment of cancer involves surgery, radiotherapy, and chemotherapy. Chemotherapy involves the use of synthetic and natural origin drugs in proper doses for a certain period of time [64]. Chemotherapy causes severe adverse effects in pateints, either synthetic or natural origin drugs, that's why we need to develop new, safer chemotherapeutic agents from natural products. Several medicinal plants such as berberis, zinger, garlic, olives, neem, *etc*. show cytotoxic activities in preclinical trials should be evaluated in clinical trials to develop new phytochemicals for this deadly disease [65 - 69]. Over 53% of the current anticancer drugs were derived in one way or another from natural sources. In this section of the book chapter, we summarized natural products with anticancer activity.

3.1. Bioactive Phytochemicals with Anticancer Activity

3.1.1. Vincristine and Vinblastine

Vincristine and vinblastine Fig. (**8**) are belonging to indole alkaloids and isolated from aerial parts of periwinkle (*Vinca rosea* or *Catharanthus roseus*, Apocynaceae). This plant is usually grown as an ornamental plant. Eli Lilly pharmaceutical company developed this anticancer medicine and successfully utilized in cancer treatment [70 - 72].

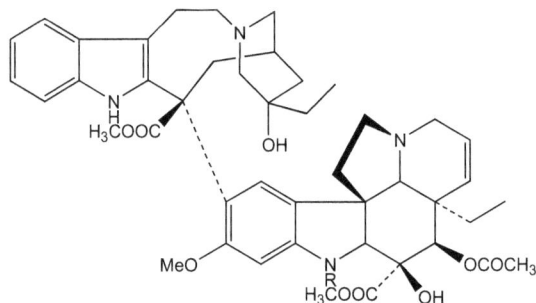

Fig. (8). Chemical structure of Vincristine R = CH₃;Vinblastine R = CHO.

3.1.2. Podophyllotoxins

Podophyllotoxins were isolated from *Podophyllum peltatum* L. and *P. emodii* Wallich (Berberidaceae). Traditionally this plant is used for the treatment of skin diseases. In 1980, podophyllotoxin was isolated, but in the 1950s it developed as an anticancer agent [69]. Several clinical trials failed to establish it as anticancer agent due to its efficacy and unacceptable toxicity. The first derivatives of podophyllotoxin, etoposide (Fig. **9**), and then teniposide were clinically proven and developed as anticancer agents. Etoposide and teniposide are used for the treatment of lymphomas, bronchial, and testicular cancers [73].

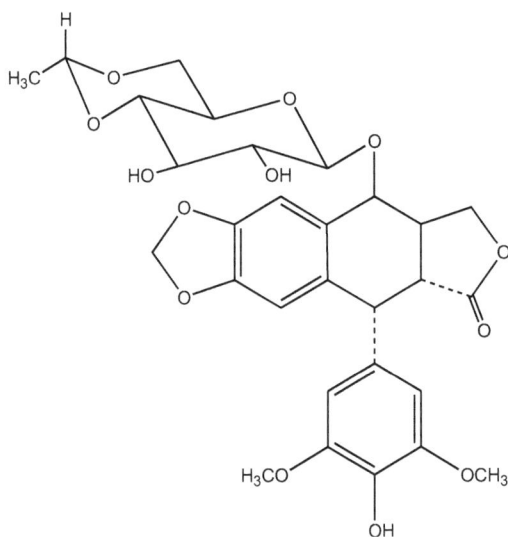

Fig. (9). Chemical structure of Etoposide.

3.1.3. Taxanes

Taxanes are complex organic compounds obtained from Taxus sp. (*Taxus brevifolia* and *T. baccata*, Taxaceae). Taxanes are discovered by the NCI program of screening of anticancer chemicals from plants [69]. Paclitaxel Fig. (**10**) isolated from *T. brevifolia* and docetaxel, a semisynthetic derivative from 10-deacetylbaccatin III (DAB) was isolated from leaves of *T. baccata*. Paclitaxel is used for the treatment of breast, ovarian, and non-small cell lung cancer while docetaxel is used for the treatment of breast and non-small cell lung cancer [74, 75].

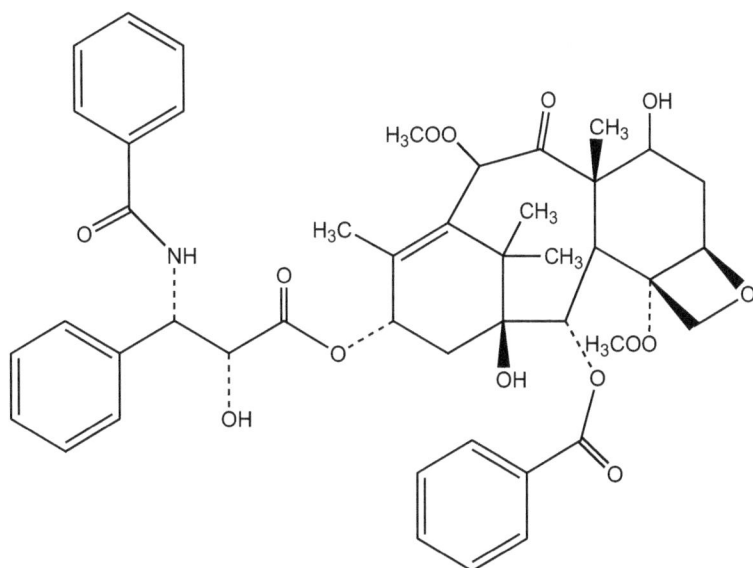

Fig. (10). Chemical structure of Paclitaxel.

3.1.4. Camptothecins

Camptothecins Fig. (**11**) are quinoline alkaloids isolated from *Camptotheca acuminata* Decne (Nyssaceae). In China, it is grown as an ornamental plant. Topotecan, irinotecan, and semisynthetic derivatives of camptothecins were developed by an extensive research [76]. Cositecan and silatecan are also lipophilic semisynthetic derivatives of camptothecins [77]. Several water-soluble salts of camptothecin, such as elemotecan, lurtotecan, and namitecan, are in clinical development [78].

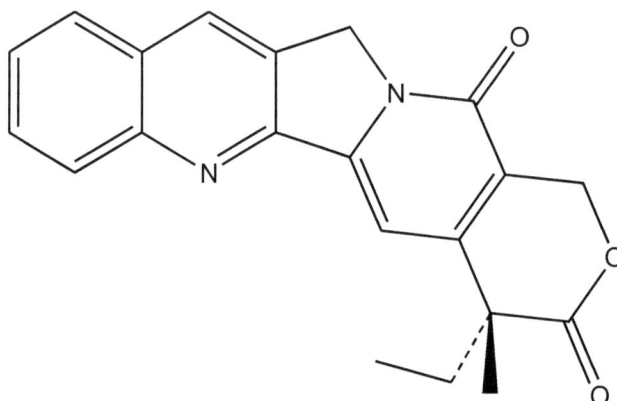

Fig. (11). Chemical structure of Camptothecin.

3.1.5. Colchicine

Colchicine Fig. (**12**) was isolated from seed and corm of the *Colchicum autumnale* and *C. luteum* (Liliaceae). Colchicine is an amorphous, yellowish-white alkaloid [69]. Demecolcine, also a constituent of *Colchicum*, is a more immediate precursor of colchicine. This alkaloid is also used in biological experiments to produce polyploidy or multiplication of the chromosomes in a cell nucleus. Such properties make it suitable for use in horticulture and cultivation of medicinal plants. Colchicine significantly reduces incident cancer in Gout male patients. Recent studies showed antitumor activity of colchicine [79].

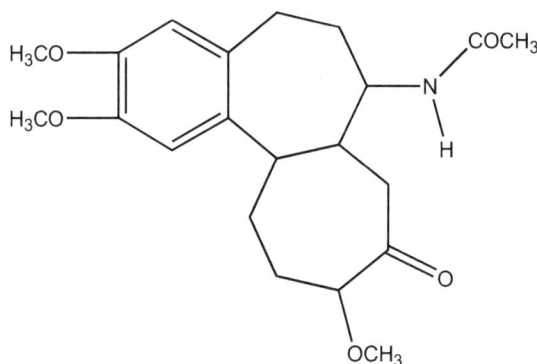

Fig. (12). Chemical structure of Colchicine.

3.1.6. Resveratrol

Resveratrol Fig. (**13**) was isolated from red wine and also reported from several natural sources. Resveratrol is a phenolic compound with tremendous antioxidant activity. Recent preclinical and clinical studies have shown its beneficial effect in the treatment of cancer. Resveratrol primarily inhibits skin carcinogenesis by a pleiotropic mechanism [80]. Currently, around 15,800 research papers were published in the scientific journals related to resveratrol, and around 6,700 papers only related to cancer [81]. That makes resveratrol a promising candidate in the drug discovery cascade of anticancer agents. Bioactive natural products with antitumor and cytotoxic activities are summarized in Table **3**.

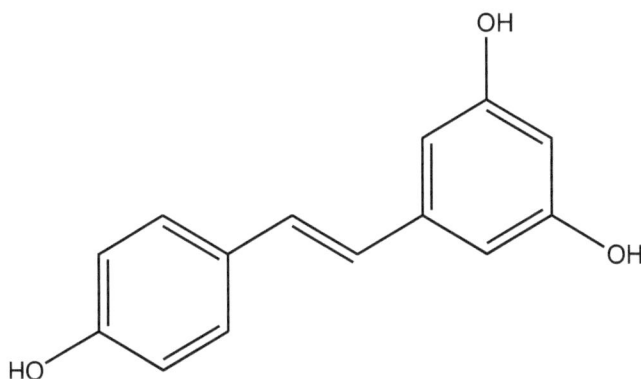

Fig. (13). Chemical structure of *trans*-Resveratrol.

Table 3. Bioactive phytochemicals with anticancer activity.

Phytochemicals	Source	Pharmacological Action	References
Alexin B, Emodin	*Aloe vera*	Stomach cancer, neuroectodermal cancer, and leukemia	[82]
Allylmercaptocysteine, allicin	*Allium sativum*	Colon cancer, bladder carcinoma	[83]
Asiatic acid	*Centella asiatica*	Daltons lymphoma, breast cancer, and melanoma	[84]
Berberine	*Berberis vulgaris*	Breast, prostate, and leukemia	[85]
Boswellic acid	*Boswellia serrata*	Prostate cancer	[86]
β-Caryophyllene, α-zingiberene	*Peristrophe bicalyculata*	MCF7, MDA-MB-468	[87]
Colchicine	*Colchicum autumnale*	Hodgkin's lymphoma, chronic granulocytic leukemia	[79]
Curcumin	*Curcuma longa*	Breast, lung, liver, prostate and skin cancers	[88]
Genistein and daidzein	*Glycine max*	Breast cancer, uterus, cervix, lung and stomach cancers	[89]
Epicatechin	*Litchi cinensis*	MCF7	[90]

Phytochemicals	Source	Pharmacological Action	References
Ginkgolides	*Ginkgo biloba*	Hepatocarcinoma, prostate, liver, and glioblastoma	[91]
Nimbolide	*Azadirachta indica*	Lymphoma, melanoma, leukemia and prostate cancer	[92]
Panaxadiol and panaxatriol	*Panax ginseng*	Breast, ovary, lung and colon cancers	[93]
Piperine, piperidine	*Piper nigrum*	B16F10 (melanoma)	[94]
Podophyllotoxins, etoposide and teniposide	*Podophyllum hexandrum*	Breast, ovary, lung, liver, brain cancers and Hodgkin's disease	[95]
Psoralidin	*Psoralea corylifolia*	Stomach and prostate cancer	[96]
Solasonine and solamargine	*Solanum nigrum*	Breast, liver and lung cancers	[97]
Thymoquinone	*Nigella sativa*	Breast, cervix, lung, GIT, thyroid cancers	[99]
Oleanolic acid and ursolic acid	*Prunella vulgaris*	Breast, cervix, lung cancers and leukemia.	[99]
Vincristine and vinblastine	*Vinca rosea*	Breast, ovary, lung, testis cancers and lymphoma, Hodgkin's disease	[72]
Withaferins	*Withania somnifera*	Cervix, prostate, colon and breast cancers	[100]

4.   HERBAL   MEDICINES   WITH   ANTI-INFLAMMATORY   AND ANTIOXIDANT POTENTIAL

Inflammation is the pathophysiological response of vascular tissues to damaging living tissue, for example, pathogens, harmed cells, or augmentations. It is a protective attempt by the living being to expel the damaging improvements just as a start the recovering procedure for the tissue [101]. Inflammation is not an analogous word for contamination since the disease is caused by an exogenous pathogen, whereas irritation is the organism's response to the pathogen. Without inflammation, the wounds and diseases could never heal, and complex tissue degradation would reduce the organism's strength. Nevertheless, untreated discomfort may also cause a wide number of diseases, such as rheumatoid pain, fatigue, and atherosclerosis. Though it is a defensive mechanism, the body is continuously under firm regulation. Intense inflammation is a rapid procedure that is revealed by excessive signs of inflammation-expansion, redness, discomfort, warmth, and capacity loss, due to leukocyte infiltration of the tissues [102]. The procedure of deep inflammation is started by the veins' neighborhood to the harmed tissue, which adjusts to permit the exudation of plasma proteins and leukocytes into the surrounding tissue. The expanded progression of liquid into the tissue causes the trademark swelling related Intense inflammation, and the expanded blood vessels in the area cause the reddened colour and prolonged warmth. The blood vessels likewise change to allow the extravasation of leukocytes through the endothelium cells and basement film covering the blood vessel. Once in the tissue, the cells move along a chemotactic slope to arrive at the site of damage, where they can effort to expel the improvement and repair the tissue [103, 104]. Chronic inflammation is an obsessed condition described by simultaneous dynamic irritation, tissue demolition, and endeavors at repair. Chronic inflammation isn't exposed by the classic signs of acute inflammation recorded previously. Rather, chronically inflamed tissue is rendered by the penetration of monocytes, macrophages, lymphocytes and plasma cells, tissue destruction, and events at healing, which combine angiogenesis and fibrosis. Endogenous causes integrate persistent acute inflammation while exogenous causes are altered and integrate bacterial disease, particularly by Mycobacterium tuberculosis, delayed exposure to synthetic agents, for example, silica, or immune system responses (rheumatoid joint inflammation) [102]. In acute inflammation, exclusion of the advancement stops the enrolment of monocytes into the inflamed tissue, and current macrophages leave tissue through the lymphatics.

4.1. Current Therapies for Inflammation

Anti-inflammatory agents are substances used to reduce inflammation. Anti-inflammatory drugs also behave as analgesics, by reducing inflammation as opposed to opioids, which affect the brain. They are of two kinds: steroidal anti-inflammatory drugs and non -steroidal anti-inflammatory drugs. Steroidal anti-inflammatory drugs reduce inflammation by binding to cortisol receptors. These drugs are referred to as corticosteroids. Non-steroidal anti-inflammatory drugs (NSAIDs) reduce pain by inhibiting the cyclooxygenase (COX) enzyme involved in prostaglandin synthesis [101, 105].

4.2. Bioactive Phytochemicals with Anti-inflammatory and Antioxidant Activity

The side effects of anti-inflammatory drugs are the main problems of modern medicine today. Therefore, the development of new and more powerful anti-inflammatory drugs with lesser side effects is wanted. In addition to standard drugs, many herbal plants have anti-inflammatory effects such as turmeric, ginger, willow bark, garlic, and hyssop, *etc*. Rheumatoid arthritis is an autoimmune disease considered by chronic inflammation, hyper-proliferation of the synovial lining, and cartilage demolition. Anti-inflammatory drugs, presently available for the treatment of inflammation of various diseases, have unwanted side effects such as peptic ulcers [106 - 108]. Therefore, plant formulation and traditional preparations have become progressively popular and are regularly chosen over synthetically derived pharmaceuticals. Although many herbal plant extracts have been clinically used as anti-inflammatory remedies in the treatment of inflammation, gouty, rheumatoid arthritis, their mode of action remains unclear [106]. The interface between the compounds from herbal plants and the diseased state of rheumatism might be far more complicatedthan merely the result of an anti-inflammatory activity used by a single bioactive molecule or a group of isolated phytomedicine. So, discovering and regulating the good combination of anti-inflammatory herbal plants available in the Indian system of medicine holds the key in declining the sufferings of human beings from this painful disease, rheumatoid arthritis. Table **4** compiles the bioactive phytochemicals with anti-inflammatory and antioxidant properties (Fig. **14**).

Table 4. Bioactive phytochemicals with anti-inflammatory and antioxidant activity.

Phytochemicals	Source	References
β-Sistosterol, linalool, leteolingyucoside, dehydroanonaine	*Nelumbo nucifera*	[109]
Tiliroside, patuletin-3-*O*-β-*D*-glycopyranoside	*Pfaffia townsendii*	[110]
β-Pinene	*Nardostachys jatamansi*	[111]
Gallic acid, quercetin	*Polygonum odoratum*	[112]
Arjundic acid, isoprotenol, ellagic acid, betulinic acid, β-sitosterol	*Terminalia arjuna*	[113]
3,7,11,15-Tetramethyl-hxabecen-1-ol	*Alnus nitida*	[114]
Gallic acid, quercetin, kaempferol, myricetin	*Pistacia atlantica*	[115]
Apigenin, protocatechuic acid, proto-catechualdehyde, hentriacontanol, calycosin, rutin, quercetin	*Cardiospermum halicacabum*	[116]
Swertiamarin	*Enicostemma littorale*	[117]
Tannins, flavonoids alkaloids, saponins, steroids and phenolic compounds	*Corallocarpus epigeous*	[118]
Volatile fractions	*Alpinia speciosa*	[119]
Triterpenoids	*Momordica charantia*	[120]
Zingiberene, β-bisabolene, α-farnesene, β-sesquiphellandrene, and α-curcumene	*Zingiber officinale*	[121]
Flavonoid	*Allium sativum*	[122]
Bacopasaponins A-G, bacopaside I-VIII, bacopaside	*Bacopa monnieri*	[123]
Protein, fat, energy, Vitamin A, E, K	*Ocimum basillicum*	[124]
Curcumin, curcumenol β-sesquiphellandrene	*Curcuma longa*	[125]
Tinosporafuranol, tinosporafurandiol, tinosporaclerodanol, β-sitosterol	*Tinospora cardifolia*	[126]
Hyperforin, pseudo-hypericin, amentoflavin	*Hypericum perforatum*	[126]
Protocatechnic acid	*Boswellia dalzielii*	[126]

(Table 4) cont.....

Phytochemicals	Source	References
Ellagic acid, arjundic acid, betulinic acid, β-sitosterol	*Dissotis thollonii*	[127]
7-Dihydroxy-4-methoxy flavones	*Gmelina arborea*	[128]

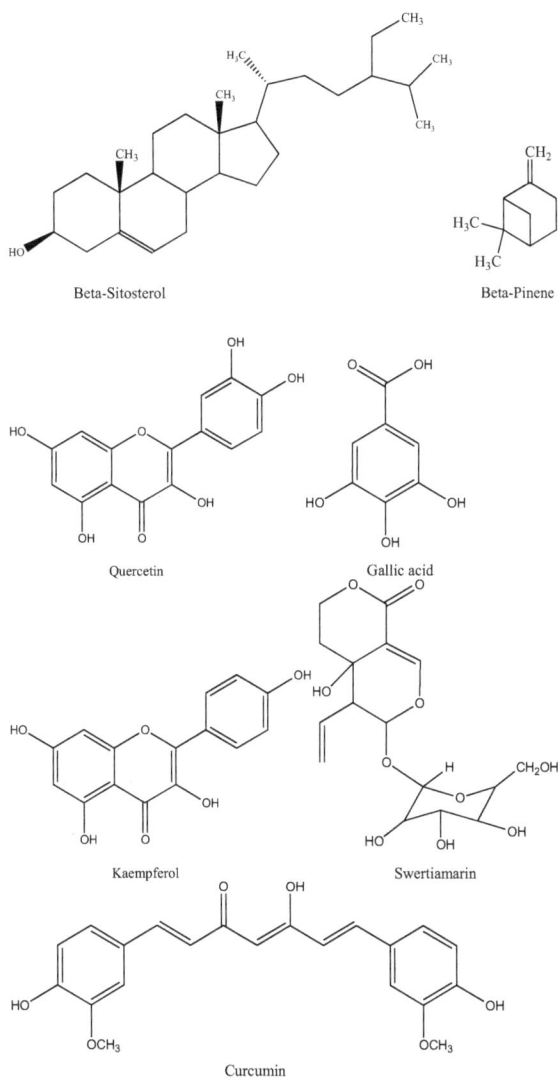

Fig. (14). Chemical structure of some bioactive phytochemical with anti-inflammatory and antioxidant activity.

5. HERBAL MEDICINES WITH CARDIOPROTECTIVE ACTIVITY

Cardiovascular disorders are the main cause of death in recent years. Coronary heart disease is the single largest killer of American males and females: American Heart Association. It is described that seven million Americans suffer from CHD, and about half a million die each year from heart attacks. Both epidemiologic and clinical trials have recognized that high levels of LDL-c and reduced levels of HDL-c are related to an amplified risk of CHD [129]. According to the National Cholesterol Education Program guidelines, all patients at least 20 years of age should have an initial cholesterol measurement. The American Diabetes Association recommends a complete lipid profile each year. In one of the studies showed by Lipid Research Clinics, Coronary Primary Prevention Trial reported that 11% reduction in LDL-c was associated with a 19% reduction in CHD risk.

Further, Helsinki Heart Study validated a significant reduction in CHD events among diabetes cases by the management of hypercholesterolemia. A number of pieces of evidence are available showing the reduction in risk for CHD by acceptable management of dyslipidaemia among diabetic patients. Lipoprotein (a) and homocysteine are two important independent risk factors for coronary artery disease. Each one plays an important role in the development of atherosclerosis through effects on thrombolysis, the endothelium, and platelets. Lipoprotein (a) is an acute phase reactant and has a strong association with IL-6 pro-inflammatory marker. Lipoprotein (a) binds endothelial cells, macrophages, fibroblasts, and platelets;these may promote the proliferation of vascular smooth muscle cells and affect human monocytes [130]. There is evidence that c-reactive protein (CRP) has a role in the pathogenesis of atherosclerosis. In this process, CRP is markedly up-regulated in atheromatous plaques.CRP may promote low-density lipoprotein cholesterol uptake by macrophages, and may also induce the expression of intercellular adhesion molecules by endothelial cells.

The goal of lipid-lowering involvement is to prevent the onset of CHD and also escaping CHD events. These involvements include lifestyle modification like diet, exercise, and smoking cessation, including pharmacologic measures. A reduction in fatty substances and cholesterol in the diet, as well as regular physical activities, are two essential lifestyle modifications [131]. Thus, physical activity, along with weight reduction, has reflected to be an essential component in the management of elevated cholesterol levels. Drug therapy is mostly measured for the adult patient who has LDL-c 190 mg/dl or greater without two other risk factors. It is observed that certain cultural food habits are responsible for dyslipidaemia, which makes it more life-threatening for the people already suffering from dyslipideamia. The most important risk factors contributing to the progress of CHD diseases. Raised levels of cholesterol, LDL, and triglycerides in diabetes have been specified as major risk factors for CHD. The most common health problem in obese singles include hypertension, Type II diabetcs, hyperlipidaemia, coronary artery disease, gastrointestinal disease, peripheral vascular disease, and also certain types of cancer. Obese individuals with excess abdominal or visceral fatty have a higher risk of metabolic syndrome X. Statins are the most commonly used agents for dyslipidaemia. Moreover, controlling dyslipidaemia statins also have a strong plaque stabilizing effect, which decreases the incidence of acute coronary events [132, 133]. According to the expert panel of research, evaluation and treatment of high blood cholesterol in adults, long term application of statin causes gastrointestinal discomfort. However, amongst the various lipid lowering agents, like nicotinic acid, fibric acid derivatives, and statins, statin is the drug of choice in the management of dyslipidaemia. Statins are the leading agent presenting anti-proliferative, anti-inflammatory, antioxidant, anti-platelet effects, and having the ability to prolong the half-life of endothelial cells. Sibutramin and orlistat, both the drugs are accepted for obesity management by the FDA, but its long term use is not safe and cause mood enhancement and cardiovascular excitation [133]. Recent data recommended that statin therapy based on C- reactive protein (CRP) values would result in few events and relapse of atherosclerosis [134].

5.1. Current Therapies for Treatment of Cardiovascular Diseases

Current drugs available for the management of cardiovascular diseases are not ideal and having severe adverse effects. Plant-based drug has been validated in the management of atherosclerosis, dyslipidemia, obesity, *etc.*, such as *Dioscorea bulbifera, Terminalia arjuna, Curcuma longa, Bacopa monnieri, Hippophae rahmnoidse and Salacia reticulataetc*. Their anti-obesity, hypoglycaemic and hypolipidemic effects are stated in various preclinical and clinical studies.

5.1. Medicinal Plants and Bioactive Phytochemicals for Treatment of Cardiovascular Diseases

Commiphora mukul: commonly known as *Guggul,* belongs to family Burseraceae, is a highly valued medicinal plant used in theAyurveda system for controlling obesity and cholesterol. Guggul-lipid is the active chemical constituentisolated from guggul, decreases the total cholesterol, LDL-c, triglycerides as well as improves HDL-c to LDL-c ratio. *C. mukul* also has antioxidant property as it reduces lipid peroxidase. Several clinical, as well as experimental studies, have proven the hypocholesterolemic property of *C. mukul* [135].

Terminalia arjuna: commonly known as Arjuna. *Terminalia arjuna* has been prescribed as cardioprotective drug indicating its anti-atherosclerotic property. Several experimental and clinical pieces of evidence have proved the anti-atherosclerotic property of arjuna, thereby reducing the incidence of atherosclerosis and the associated cardiovascular complications. In a study, Saravanan *et al.*, found that arjuna reduced the total cholesterol and HDL-cholesterol ratio among the experimental animals indicating its lipid-lowering property. He also observed a marked reduction in total cholesterol among the cholesterol-fed rabbits. *T. arjuna* also reduced the triglycerides and elevated the high-density lipoproteins among the treated group of rabbits [136].

Tribulus terrestris: also known as Gokshur. Diosgenin, gitogenin, chlorogenin, kaempferol,3-glucoside, 3-rutinoside, and tribuloside are major compounds isolated from fruit and leaves of *T. terrestris*. The plant *T. terrestris* is one of the ingredients of present test formulation, used for the treatment of arterial blood pressure and has cardiac stimulant action [137].

Bacopa monnieri: a family of the Scrophulariaceae, is a small, crawling herb and cultivates naturally in wet soil, shallow water, and swamps. The entire plant is utilized therapeutically. Phytocompounds responsible for the pharmacological effects of *Bacopa* include alkaloids, steroids, and saponins. Numerous bioactive constituents such as brahmine and herpestine, d-mannitol, and hersaponin acid A and monnierin were isolated in India more than 40 years earlier. Other dynamic constituents have been documented, including stigmasterol, beta sitosterol, betulic acid, stigmasterol, bacosides, and bacopasaponins [138].

Hippophae rhamnoides: This fruit belongs to Elaeagnaceae family and scattered over Asia and Europe. Various parts of *H. rhamnoides* have been utilized for the treatment of ailments in traditional medicine in various countries. It contains a series of bioactive molecules with tocopherols, lipids, sterols, ascorbic acid, tannins, and carotenoids. However, flavonoids are invented to be its most active bioactive molecules. These lead molecules possess natural and therapeutic activity, including cardioprotective anticancer, antitumor, antioxidant, immunomodulatory, and hepato-protective properties. *H. rhamnoides,* a high-altitude plant thatcontains folic acid along with B6, B12 is engaged to validate its valuable role in reducing the homocysteine level with the purpose of diminishing the risk of CHD [139]. In Table **5**, we summarized bioactive phytochemical accountable for cardio protective activities (Fig. **15**).

Table 5. Bioactive phytochemicals responsible for Cardio protective activity.

Phytoconstituents	Source	References
Triterperoid saponin, arjunolic acid, arjunogenin, arjunine, myricetin, quercetin, kaemferol	*Terminalia arjuna*	[140]
Momordenol, momordicin, momordicinin charantidiol	*Momordica charantia*	[141]
Allicin	*Allium sativum*	[142, 143]

(Table 5) cont.....

Phytoconstituents	Source	References
Glycyrrhizin, glycyrrhetinic acid	*Glycyrrhiza glabra*	[144]
Sesquiterpenes, flavanoids	*Saussurea lappa*	[145]
Alkaloids, saponins, carvone, thymol, myristic acid	*Nigella sativa*	[146]
Gallic acid, phenolic compounds, rosemarinic acid	*Ocimum basilicum*	[147]
Cinnamaldehyde, eugenol, phellandrene, mono and sesquiterpenes	*Cinnamomum tamala*	[148]
Vitamin A, B 12, triterpenoid curcubitacins B, lageninin	*Lagenaria siceraria*	[149]
Caffeic acid	*Raphanus sativus*	[150]
Columbin, palmarin and tinosporic acid	*Tinospora cordifolia*	[151]
Mangiferin	*Mangifera indica*	[152]
Methyl-n-heptanoa,1-octanoate,n-Nananoic acid, *n*-tridecanoic	*Tamarindus indica*	[153]
Digoxin, digitoxin, gitoxin, gitaloxin, glygogetaloxin	*Digitalis purpurea*	[121]
Zingiberene, phellandrene, gingerol and shagoal	*Zingiber officinale*	[154]
Apigenin, rosameric acid and eugenol	*Ocimum sanctum*	[155]
Tropane alkaloids	*Datura fastuosa*	[156]

6. HERBAL MEDICINES WITH ANTIOBESITY ACTIVITY

Obesity is a serious illness that triggers a variety of severe human diseases such as cardiovascular complications and diabetes mellitus. These cardiovascular complications have emerged as the top killer for humans worldwide. Obesity nowadaysisconsidered as the '*New World Syndrome*'. WHO defined obesity as *a condition of abnormal or excessive fat accumulation in adipose tissue, to the extent that health may be impaired.* The prevalence of obesity has increased dramatically in the last decade, from 12 to 20% in men and from 16 to 25% in females worldwide [157 - 159]. Traditionally natural products and medicinal plants were used for controlling obesity and related complications.

6.1. Current Strategies for Management of Obesity

Limited drug therapies are available for the management of obesity; only sibutramine and orlistat are approved from the US FDA for long term use. Medicinal plants traditionally also reported to have weight reduction properties such as fennel, ocimum, ginger, trigonella, garlic *etc*. Lifestyle management, exercise, diet control also helps in controlling obesity [160, 161].

Arjunolic acid

Gallic acid

Digitoxigenin

Gitoxigenin

Quercetin

Kaempferol

phanthidin

O-rhamnose-glucose

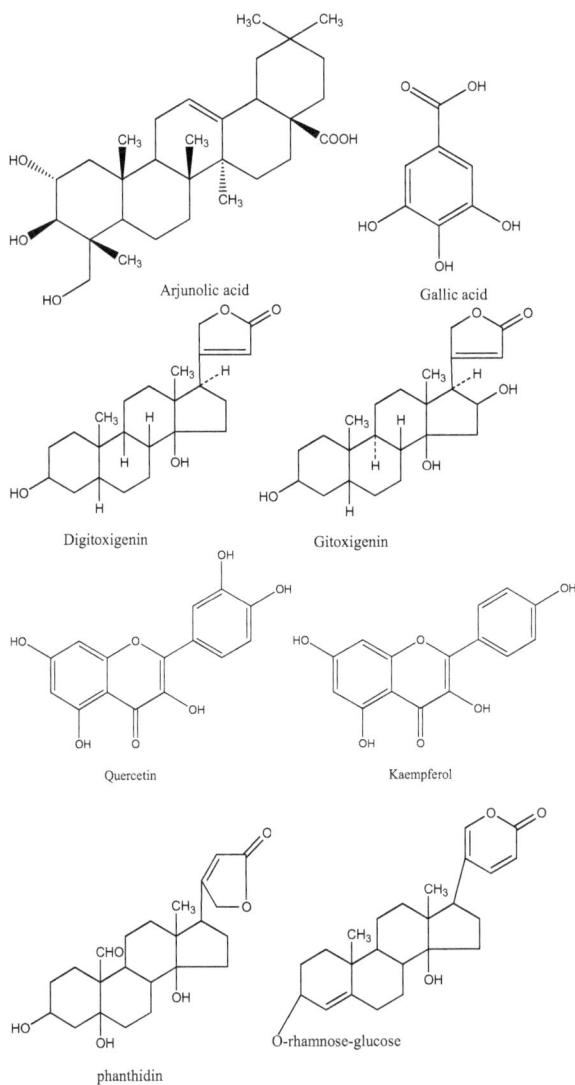

Fig. (15). Chemical structure of some bioactive phytochemical responsible to Cardio protective activity.

6.2. Role of Herbal Medicines for the Treatment of Obesity

In modern medicine, there is no single drug that reduces obesity without serious adverse effects, that is why nowadays people prefer to use medicinal plants and herbal remedies for controlling obesity. Modern drugs derived from natural products or herbal drugs playan essential role in the treatment of human ailments [162 - 164]. Table **6** summarizes bioactive phytochemicals and medicinal plant extracts with anti-obesity effects (Fig. **16**).

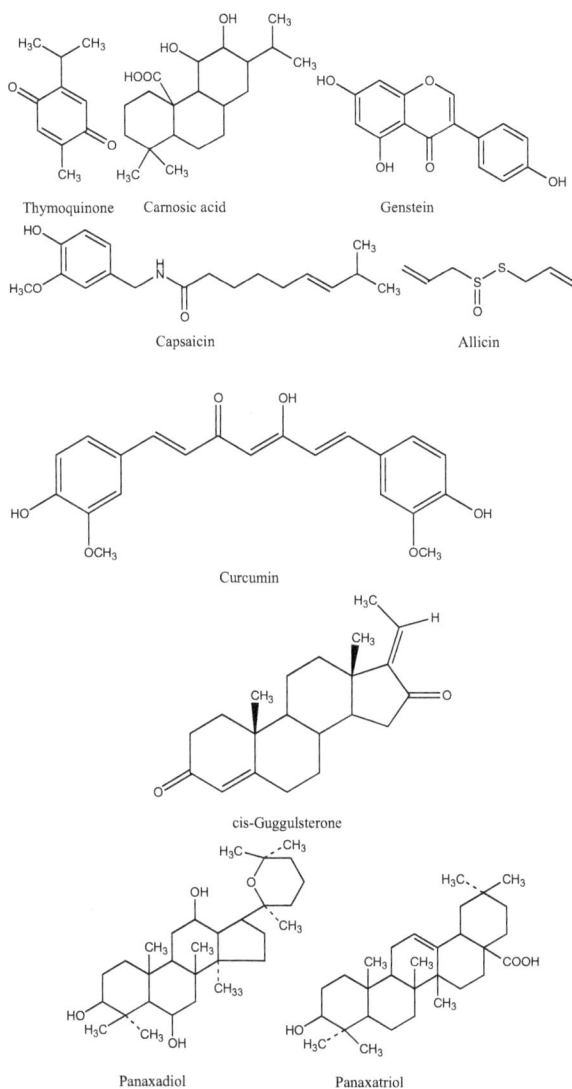

Fig. (**16**). Chemical structure of some bioactive phytochemicals with antiobesity activity.

Table 6. Bioactive phytochemicals with anti-obesity activity.

Phytochemicals	Source	References
Thymoquinone	*Nigella sativa* L.	[165]
(-)-Epigallocatechin gallate	*Thea sinensis* L.	[166]
Carnosic acid	*Salvia officinalis* L.	[168]

(Table 6) cont.....

Phytochemicals	Source	References
(-)-Hydroxycitric acid	*Garcina cambogia*	[169]
Genistein	*Glycine max* L.	[169]
Capsaicin	*Capsicum annuum* L.	[169]
Ellagitannins	*Lagerstroemia speciosa* L.	[169]
Ginsenosides	*Panax ginseng*	[169]
Silibinin	*Silybum marianum* L.	[169]
Allicin	*Allium sativum* L.	[169]
Curcumin	*Curcuma longa* L.	[169]
cis-Guggulsterone	*Commiphora mukul*	[169]

CONCLUDING REMARKS

Medicinal plants are a major source of drug discovery. Natural products are considered safe based on their long history of use as food by humans. Plants are considered as an unlimited source of novel and complex compounds that most likely would never be the target of an early synthetic program, *e.g.*, artemisinin, quinine, morphine, vinblastine, vincristine, taxol, and digoxin *etc*. Due to recent advances in the field of extraction, isolation, characterization, and pharmacological screening methods, natural products become good candidates for drug discovery and development.

ABBREVIATIONS

BMI   Body mass index

CHD   Coronary heart disease

COX   Cyclooxygenase

DPP-IV   Dipeptidyl peptidase IV inhibitors

DM   Diabetes mellitus

DLA   Dalton's lymphoma ascites

EAC   Ehrlich ascites carcinoma

NSAIDs Non-steroidal anti-inflammatory drugs

NSCLC   Non-small cell lung cancer

SGLTi's Sodium dependent glucose transporter inhibitors

WHO   World health organization

CONSENT FOR PUBLICATION

Not applicable.

CONFLICT OF INTEREST

The author(s) confirms that there is no conflict of interest.

ACKNOWLEDGEMENTS

Declared none.

REFERENCES

[1]   Ahamad J, Toufeeq I, Khan MA, *et al.* Oleuropein: A natural antioxidant molecule in the treatment of metabolic syndrome. Phytother Res 2019; 33(12): 3112-28.
        [http://dx.doi.org/10.1002/ptr.6511] [PMID: 31746508]

[2]   Fabricant DS, Farnsworth NR. The value of plants used in traditional medicine for drug discovery. Environ Health Perspect 2001; 109(1) (Suppl. 1): 69-75.
        [PMID: 11250806]

[3]   Dubey NK, Kumar R, Tripathi P. Global promotion of herbal medicine: India's opportunity. Current Med 2004; 86: 37-41.

[4]   Grover JK, Yadav S, Vats V. Medicinal plants of India with anti-diabetic potential. J Ethnopharmacol 2002; 81(1): 81-100.
        [http://dx.doi.org/10.1016/S0378-8741(02)00059-4] [PMID: 12020931]

[5]   Ahamad J, Hasan N, Amin S, Mir SR. Swertiamarin contributes to glucose homeostasis *via* inhibition of carbohydrate metabolizing enzymes. J Nat Rem 2016; 16(4): 125-30.
        [http://dx.doi.org/10.18311/jnr/2016/7634]

[6]   Ahamad J, Naquvi KJ, Mir SR, Ali M. Review on role of natural alpha-glucosidase inhibitors for management of diabetes mellitus. Int J Biomed Res 2011; 6: 374-80.

[7]   Newman DJ, Cragg GM. Natural products as sources of new drugs from 1981 to 2014. J Nat Prod 2016; 79(3): 629-61.
        [http://dx.doi.org/10.1021/acs.jnatprod.5b01055] [PMID: 26852623]

[8]   Bell GI. Lilly lecture 1990. Molecular defects in diabetes mellitus. Diabetes 1991; 40(4): 413-22.
        [http://dx.doi.org/10.2337/diab.40.4.413] [PMID: 2010042]

[9]   Sowers JR, Epstein M, Frohlich ED. Diabetes, hypertension, and cardiovascular disease: an update. Hypertension 2001; 37(4): 1053-9.
        [http://dx.doi.org/10.1161/01.HYP.37.4.1053] [PMID: 11304502]

[10]   Giugliano D, Ceriello A, Paolisso G. Diabetes mellitus, hypertension, and cardiovascular disease: which role for oxidative stress? Metabolism 1995; 44(3): 363-8.
        [http://dx.doi.org/10.1016/0026-0495(95)90167-1] [PMID: 7885282]

[11]   Bailey CJ, Day C. Traditional plant medicines as treatments for diabetes. Diabetes Care 1989; 12(8): 553-64.
        [http://dx.doi.org/10.2337/diacare.12.8.553] [PMID: 2673695]

[12]   The pharmacological basis of therapeutics. 10th ed. McGraw-Hill Medical Publishing division, New Delhi, India. Allahabad, India 2001; pp. 89-1689.

[13]   Alarcon-Aguilara FJ, Roman-Ramos R, Perez-Gutierrez S, Aguilar-Contreras A, Contreras-Weber CC,

Flores-Saenz JL. Study of the anti-hyperglycemic effect of plants used as antidiabetics. J Ethnopharmacol 1998; 61(2): 101-10.
[http://dx.doi.org/10.1016/S0378-8741(98)00020-8] [PMID: 9683340]

[14]   Ahamad J, Amin S, Mir SR. *Momordica charantia:* Review on Phytochemistry and Pharmacology. Res J Phytochem 2017; 11: 53-65.
[http://dx.doi.org/10.3923/rjphyto.2017.53.65]

[15]   Lotlikar MM, Rao R. Pharmacology of a hypoglycaemic principle isolated from the fruits of *Momordica charantia* Linn. Indian J Pharm 1966; 28(5): 129-33.

[16]   Handa G, Singh J, Sharma ML, Kaul A, Zafar R. Hypoglycaemic principle of *Momordica charantia* seeds. Indian J Nat Prod 1990; 6(1): 16-9.

[17]   Khanna P, Jain SC, Panagariya A, Dixit VP. Hypoglycemic activity of polypeptide-p from a plant source. J Nat Prod 1981; 44(6): 648-55.
[http://dx.doi.org/10.1021/np50018a002] [PMID: 7334382]

[18]   Nhiem NX, Kiem PV, Minh CV, *et al.* α-Glucosidase inhibition properties of cucurbitane-type triterpene glycosides from the fruits of *Momordica charantia.* Chem Pharm Bull (Tokyo) 2010; 58(5): 720-4.
[http://dx.doi.org/10.1248/cpb.58.720] [PMID: 20460803]

[19]   Yibchok-anun S, Adisakwattana S, Yao CY, Sangvanich P, Roengsumran S, Hsu WH. Slow acting protein extract from fruit pulp of *Momordica charantia* with insulin secretagogue and insulinomimetic activities. Biol Pharm Bull 2006; 29(6): 1126-31.
[http://dx.doi.org/10.1248/bpb.29.1126] [PMID: 16755004]

[20]   Xu X, Shan B, Liao C-H, Xie J-H, Wen P-W, Shi J-Y. Anti-diabetic properties of *Momordica charantia* L. polysaccharide in alloxan-induced diabetic mice. Int J Biol Macromol 2015; 81: 538-43.
[http://dx.doi.org/10.1016/j.ijbiomac.2015.08.049] [PMID: 26318666]

[21]   Hassan N, Ahamad J, Amin S, Mir SR. Rapid preparative isolation of erythrocentaurin from *Enicostemma littorale* by medium pressure liquid chromatography, its estimation by a validated HPTLC densitometric method and α-amylase inhibitory activity. J Sep Sci 2015; 38(4): 592-8.
[http://dx.doi.org/10.1002/jssc.201401030] [PMID: 25504557]

[22]   Dhanavathy G. Immunohistochemistry, histopathology, and biomarker studies of swertiamarin, a secoiridoid glycoside, prevents and protects streptozotocin-induced β-cell damage in Wistar rat pancreas. J Endocrinol Invest 2015; 38(6): 669-84.
[http://dx.doi.org/10.1007/s40618-015-0243-5] [PMID: 25770453]

[23]   Vaidya HB, Ahmed AA, Goyal RK, Cheema SK. Glycogen phosphorylase-a is a common target for anti-diabetic effect of iridoid and secoiridoid glycosides. J Pharm Pharm Sci 2013; 16(4): 530-40.
[http://dx.doi.org/10.18433/J3FS4F] [PMID: 24210061]

[24]   Alkefai NH, Ahamad J, Amin S, Mir SR. Arylated gymnemic acids from *Gymnema sylvestre* R.Br. as potential α-glucosidase inhibitors. Phytochem Lett 2018; 25: 196-02.
[http://dx.doi.org/10.1016/j.phytol.2018.04.021]

[25]   Alkefai NH, Sharma M, Ahamad J, Amin S, Mir SR. New olean-15-ene type gymnemic acids from *Gymnema sylvestre* (Retz.) R.Br. and their antihyperglycemic activity through α-glucosidase inhibition. Phytochem Lett 2019; 32: 83-9.
[http://dx.doi.org/10.1016/j.phytol.2019.05.005]

[26]   Fushiki T, Kojima A, Imoto T, Inoue K, Sugimoto E. An extract of *Gymnema sylvestre* leaves and purified gymnemic acid inhibits glucose-stimulated gastric inhibitory peptide secretion in rats. J Nutr 1992; 122(12): 2367-73.
[http://dx.doi.org/10.1093/jn/122.12.2367] [PMID: 1453221]

[27]   Sugihara Y, Nojima H, Matsuda H, Murakami T, Yoshikawa M, Kimura I. Antihyperglycemic effects of gymnemic acid IV, a compound derived from *Gymnema sylvestre* leaves in streptozotocin-diabetic

mice. J Asian Nat Prod Res 2000; 2(4): 321-7.
[http://dx.doi.org/10.1080/10286020008041372] [PMID: 11249615]

[28] Abaza L, Taamalli A, Nsir H, Zarrouk M. A, Taamalli H, Zarrouk NM. Olive Tree (*Olea europeae* L.) leaves: importance and advances in the analysis of phenolic compounds. Antioxidants 2015; 4(4): 682-98.
[http://dx.doi.org/10.3390/antiox4040682] [PMID: 26783953]

[29] Khalili A, Nekooeian AA, Khosravi MB. Oleuropein improves glucose tolerance and lipid profile in rats with simultaneous renovascular hypertension and type 2 diabetes. J Asian Nat Prod Res 2017; 19(10): 1011-21.
[http://dx.doi.org/10.1080/10286020.2017.1307834] [PMID: 28347166]

[30] Nekooeian AA, Khalili A, Khosravi MB. Effects of oleuropein in rats with simultaneous type 2 diabetes and renal hypertension: a study of antihypertensive mechanisms. J Asian Nat Prod Res 2014; 16(9): 953-62.
[http://dx.doi.org/10.1080/10286020.2014.924510] [PMID: 24954237]

[31] Fujiwara Y, Tsukahara C, Ikeda N, *et al.* Oleuropein improves insulin resistance in skeletal muscle by promoting the translocation of GLUT4. J Clin Biochem Nutr 2017; 61(3): 196-202.
[http://dx.doi.org/10.3164/jcbn.16-120] [PMID: 29203961]

[32] Lepore SM, Morittu VM, Celano M, *et al.* Oral Administration of Oleuropein and its semisynthetic peracetylated derivative prevents hepatic steatosis, hyperinsulinemia, and weight gain in mice fed with high fat cafeteria diet. Int J Endocrinol 2015; 2015431453
[http://dx.doi.org/10.1155/2015/431453] [PMID: 26798341]

[33] Hadrich F, Bouallagui Z, Junkyu H, Isoda H, Sayadi S. The α-glucosidase and α-amylase enzyme inhibitory of hydroxytyrosol and oleuropein. J Oleo Sci 2015; 64(8): 835-43.
[http://dx.doi.org/10.5650/jos.ess15026] [PMID: 26235001]

[34] Ahamad J, Mir SR, Naquvi KJ. Hypoglycemic activity of aqueous extract of *Berberis aristata* stems bark in STZ induced rats. Int J Pharm Pharm Sci 2012; 4(2): 473-4.

[35] Semwal BC, Shah K, Chauhan NS, Divakar K, Badhe R. Anti-diabetic activity of stem bark of *B. aristata* D.C. in alloxan induced diabetic rats. Internet Jo Pharmacol 2008; 6(1): 1-9.

[36] Xu M, Xiao Y, Yin J, *et al.* Berberine promotes glucose consumption independently of AMP-activated protein kinase activation. PLoS One 2014; 9(7)e103702
[http://dx.doi.org/10.1371/journal.pone.0103702] [PMID: 25072399]

[37] Kirtikar KR, Basu BD. Indian Medicinal plants. 2nd ed. Allahabad, India 1985; Vol. I: pp. 700-1.

[38] Toppo FA, Akhand R, Pathak AK. Pharmacological actions and potential uses of *Trigonella foenum-graecum*: a review. Asian J Pharm Clinical Res 2009; 2(4): 29-38.

[39] Khosla P, Gupta DD, Nagpal RK. Effect of *Trigonella foenum-graecum* (fenugreek) on serum lipids in normal and diabetic rats. Indian J Pharmacol 1995; 27: 89-93.

[40] Jayaweera DMA. Medicinal plant: Part III. Peradeniya, Sri Lanka: Royal Botanic Garden 1981; p. 225.

[41] Yoshikawa M, Murakami T, Komatsu H, Murakami N, Yamahara J, Matsuda H. Medicinal foodstuffs. IV. Fenugreek seed. (1): structures of trigoneosides Ia, Ib, IIa, IIb, IIIa, and IIIb, new furostanol saponins from the seeds of Indian *Trigonella foenum-graecum* L. Chem Pharm Bull (Tokyo) 1997; 45(1): 81-7.
[http://dx.doi.org/10.1248/cpb.45.81] [PMID: 9023970]

[42] Devgun M, Nanda A, Ansari SH. *Pterocarpus marsupium* Roxb. - a comprehensive review. Pharm Rev 2009; 3(6): 359-63.

[43] Ahmad F, Khalid P, Khan MM, Rastogi AK, Kidwai JR. Insulin like activity in (-) epicatechin. Acta Diabetol Lat 1989; 26(4): 291-300.

[http://dx.doi.org/10.1007/BF02624640] [PMID: 2698039]

[44] Ravi K, Ramachandran B, Subramanian S. Effect of *Eugenia Jambolana* seed kernel on antioxidant defense system in streptozotocin-induced diabetes in rats. Life Sci 2004; 75(22): 2717-31.
[http://dx.doi.org/10.1016/j.lfs.2004.08.005] [PMID: 15369706]

[45] Sheela CG, Augusti KT. Antidiabetic effects of S-allyl cysteine sulphoxide isolated from garlic *Allium sativum* Linn. Indian J Exp Biol 1992; 30(6): 523-6.
[PMID: 1506036]

[46] Matsuur H, Asakawa C, Kurimoto M, Mizutani J. Alpha-glucosidase inhibitor from the seeds of balsam pear (*Momordica charantia*) and the fruit bodies of *Grifola frondosa*. Biosci Biotechnol Biochem 2002; 66(7): 1576-8.
[http://dx.doi.org/10.1271/bbb.66.1576] [PMID: 12224646]

[47] Ahamad J, Amin S, Mir SR. Antihyperglycemic activity of charantin isolated from fruits of *Momordica charantia* Linn. Int Res J Pharm 2019; 10(1): 61-4.
[http://dx.doi.org/10.7897/2230-8407.100111]

[48] Srinivasan M, Padmanabhan M, Prince PSM. Effect of aqueous Enicostemma littorale Blume extract on key carbohydrate metabolic enzymes, lipid peroxides and antioxidants in alloxan-induced diabetic rats. J Pharm Pharmacol 2005; 57(4): 497-503.
[http://dx.doi.org/10.1211/0022357055722] [PMID: 15831211]

[49] Shanmugasundaram ERB, Gopinath KL, Radha Shanmugasundaram K, Rajendran VM. Possible regeneration of the islets of Langerhans in streptozotocin-diabetic rats given *Gymnema sylvestre* leaf extracts. J Ethnopharmacol 1990; 30(3): 265-79.
[http://dx.doi.org/10.1016/0378-8741(90)90106-4] [PMID: 2259215]

[50] Yoshikawa M, Murakami T, Kadoya M, *et al*. Medicinal foodstuffs. IX. The inhibitors of glucose absorption from the leaves of *Gymnema sylvestre* R. BR. (Asclepiadaceae): structures of gymnemosides a and b. Chem Pharm Bull (Tokyo) 1997; 45(10): 1671-6.
[http://dx.doi.org/10.1248/cpb.45.1671] [PMID: 9353896]

[51] de Bock M, Derraik JG, Brennan CM, *et al*. Olive (*Olea europaea* L.) leaf polyphenols improve insulin sensitivity in middle-aged overweight men: a randomized, placebo-controlled, crossover trial. PLoS One 2013; 8(3)e57622
[http://dx.doi.org/10.1371/journal.pone.0057622] [PMID: 23516412]

[52] Oyenihi OR, Oyenihi AB, Adeyanju AA, Oguntibeju OO. Antidiabetic effects of resveratrol: The way forward in its clinical utility JDiabRes 2016.
[http://dx.doi.org/http://dx.doi.org/10.1155/2016/9737483.]

[53] Coskun O, Kanter M, Korkmaz A, Oter S. Quercetin, a flavonoid antioxidant, prevents and protects streptozotocin-induced oxidative stress and β-cell damage in rat pancreas. Pharmacol Res 2005; 51(2): 117-23.
[http://dx.doi.org/10.1016/j.phrs.2004.06.002] [PMID: 15629256]

[54] Fu Z, Liu D. Long-term exposure to genistein improves insulin secretory function of pancreatic beta-cells. Eur J Pharmacol 2009; 616(1-3): 321-7.
[http://dx.doi.org/10.1016/j.ejphar.2009.06.005] [PMID: 19540219]

[55] Liu D, Zhen W, Yang Z, Carter JD, Si H, Reynolds KA. Genistein acutely stimulates insulin secretion in pancreatic beta-cells through a cAMP-dependent protein kinase pathway. Diabetes 2006; 55(4): 1043-50.
[http://dx.doi.org/10.2337/diabetes.55.04.06.db05-1089] [PMID: 16567527]

[56] Gandhi GR, Ignacimuthu S, Paulraj MG, Sasikumar P. Antihyperglycemic activity and antidiabetic effect of methyl caffeate isolated from Solanum torvum Swartz. fruit in streptozotocin induced diabetic rats. Eur J Pharmacol 2011; 670(2-3): 623-31.
[http://dx.doi.org/10.1016/j.ejphar.2011.09.159] [PMID: 21963451]

[57]   Gunawan-Puteri MDPT, Kawabata J. Novel α-glucosidase inhibitors from *Macaranga tanarius* leaves. Food Chem 2010; 123: 384-9.
[http://dx.doi.org/10.1016/j.foodchem.2010.04.050]

[58]   Guo H, Ling W, Wang Q, Liu C, Hu Y, Xia M. Cyanidin 3-glucoside protects 3T3-L1 adipocytes against H2O2- or TNF-α-induced insulin resistance by inhibiting c-Jun NH2-terminal kinase activation. Biochem Pharmacol 2008; 75(6): 1393-401.
[http://dx.doi.org/10.1016/j.bcp.2007.11.016] [PMID: 18179781]

[59]   Kanaujia A, Duggar R, Pannakal ST, *et al.* Insulinomimetic activity of two new gallotannins from the fruits of *Capparis moonii.* Bioorg Med Chem 2010; 18(11): 3940-5.
[http://dx.doi.org/10.1016/j.bmc.2010.04.032] [PMID: 20452777]

[60]   Lee YJ, Suh KS, Choi MC, *et al.* Kaempferol protects HIT-T15 pancreatic beta cells from 2-deoxy-D-ribose-induced oxidative damage. Phytother Res 2010; 24(3): 419-23.
[http://dx.doi.org/10.1002/ptr.2983] [PMID: 19827031]

[61]   Muraoka O, Morikawa T, Miyake S, Akaki J, Ninomiya K, Yoshikawa M. Quantitative determination of potent α-glucosidase inhibitors, salacinol and kotalanol, in *Salacia* species using liquid chromatography-mass spectrometry. J Pharm Biomed Anal 2010; 52(5): 770-3.
[http://dx.doi.org/10.1016/j.jpba.2010.02.025] [PMID: 20303690]

[62]   Tian LY, Bai X, Chen XH, Fang JB, Liu SH, Chen JC. Anti-diabetic effect of methylswertianin and bellidifolin from Swertia punicea Hemsl. and its potential mechanism. Phytomedicine 2010; 17(7): 533-9.
[http://dx.doi.org/10.1016/j.phymed.2009.10.007] [PMID: 19962285]

[63]   http://seer.cancer.gov/statfacts/html/all.html

[64]   Hong WK, Sporn MB. Recent advances in chemoprevention of cancer. Science 1997; 278(5340): 1073-7.
[http://dx.doi.org/10.1126/science.278.5340.1073] [PMID: 9353183]

[65]   Newman DJ, Cragg GM. Natural products as sources of new drugs over the 30 years from 1981 to 2010. J Nat Prod 2012; 75(3): 311-35.
[http://dx.doi.org/10.1021/np200906s] [PMID: 22316239]

[66]   Cragg GM, Newman DJ. Nature: a vital source of leads for anticancer drug development. Phytochem Rev 2009; 8: 313-31.
[http://dx.doi.org/10.1007/s11101-009-9123-y]

[67]   Cragg GM, Grothaus PG, Newman DJ. Impact of natural products on developing new anti-cancer agents. Chem Rev 2009; 109(7): 3012-43.
[http://dx.doi.org/10.1021/cr900019j] [PMID: 19422222]

[68]   Grothaus PG, Cragg GM, Newman DJ. Plant natural products in anticancer drug discovery. Curr Org Chem 2010; 14: 1781-91.
[http://dx.doi.org/10.2174/138527210792927708]

[69]   Demain AL, Vaishnav P. Natural products for cancer chemotherapy. Microb Biotechnol 2011; 4(6): 687-99.
[http://dx.doi.org/10.1111/j.1751-7915.2010.00221.x] [PMID: 21375717]

[70]   Trease and Evans, Pharmacognosy. [16]th ed., Evans WC. Saunders PublicationLondon: Elsevier 2009.

[71]   Roussi F, Gueritte F, Fahy J. The vinca alkaloids. Anticancer Agents from Natural Products. 2nd ed. Boca Raton: CRC/Taylor & Francis 2012; pp. 177-98.

[72]   Keglevich P, Hazai L, Kalaus G, *et al.* Modifications on the basic skeletons of vinblastine and vincristine. Molecules 2012; 17(5): 5893-914.
[http://dx.doi.org/10.3390/molecules17055893] [PMID: 22609781]

[73]   Lee KH, Xiao Z. Podophyllotoxins and analogs.Anticancer Agents from Natural Products. 2nd ed. Boca

Raton: CRC/Taylor & Francis 2012; pp. 95-22.

[74]   Hartwell JL. Plants Used against Cancer. Lawrence: Quarterman 1982.

[75]   Kingston DGI. Taxol and its analogs.Anticancer Agents from Natural Products. 2nd ed. Boca Raton: CRC/Taylor & Francis 2012; pp. 123-75.

[76]   Rahier NJ, Thomas CJ, Hecht SM. Camptothecin and its analogs.Anticancer Agents from Natural Products. 2nd ed. Boca Raton: CRC/Taylor & Francis 2012; pp. 5-25.

[77]   Pecorelli S, Ray-Coquard I, Tredan O, *et al.* Phase II of oral gimatecan in patients with recurrent epithelial ovarian, fallopian tube or peritoneal cancer, previously treated with platinum and taxanes. Ann Oncol 2010; 21(4): 759-65.
[http://dx.doi.org/10.1093/annonc/mdp514] [PMID: 19906760]

[78]   TrocA3niz IF, CendrA3s JM, Soto E, *et al.* Population pharmacokinetic/pharmacodynamic modeling of drug-induced adverse effects of a novel homocamptothecin analog, elomotecan (BN80927), in a Phase I dose finding study in patients with advanced solid tumors. Cancer Chemother Pharmacol 2012; 70(2): 239-50.
[http://dx.doi.org/10.1007/s00280-012-1906-y] [PMID: 22699813]

[79]   Kuo MC, Chang SJ, Hsieh MC. Colchicine significantly reduces incident cancer in Gout male patients. Medicine (Baltimore) 2015; 94(50)e1570.
[http://dx.doi.org/10.1097/MD.0000000000001570] [PMID: 26683907]

[80]   Jang M, Cai L, Udeani GO, *et al.* Cancer chemopreventive activity of resveratrol, a natural product derived from grapes. Science 1997; 275(5297): 218-20.
[http://dx.doi.org/10.1126/science.275.5297.218] [PMID: 8985016]

[81]   Park EJ, Pezzuto JM. The pharmacology of resveratrol in animals and humans. Biochim Biophys Acta 2015; 1852(6): 1071-113.
[http://dx.doi.org/10.1016/j.bbadis.2015.01.014] [PMID: 25652123]

[82]   El-Shemy HA, Aboul-Soud MA, Nassr-Allah AA, Aboul-Enein KM, Kabash A, Yagi A. Antitumor properties and modulation of antioxidant enzymes, activity by Aloe vera leaf active principles isolated *via* supercritical carbon dioxide extraction. Curr Med Chem 2010; 17(2): 129-38.
[http://dx.doi.org/10.2174/092986710790112620] [PMID: 19941474]

[83]   Ranjani R, Ayya RM. Anticancer properties of *Allium sativum*- a review. Asian J Biochem Pharm Res 2012; 3: 190-6.

[84]   Heidari M, Heidari-Vala H, Sadeghi MR, Akhondi MM. The inductive effects of *Centella asiatica* on rat spermatogenic cell apoptosis *in vivo.* J Nat Med 2012; 66(2): 271-8.
[http://dx.doi.org/10.1007/s11418-011-0578-y] [PMID: 21870191]

[85]   Pierpaoli E, Damiani E, Orlando F, *et al.* Antiangiogenic and antitumor activities of berberine derivative NAX014 compound in a transgenic murine model of HER2/neu-positive mammary carcinoma. Carcinogenesis 2015; 36(10): 1169-79.
[http://dx.doi.org/10.1093/carcin/bgv103] [PMID: 26168818]

[86]   Garg P, Deep A. Anticancer potential of boswellic acid: a mini review. Hygeia J Drugs Med 2015; 7: 18-27.

[87]   Ogunwande IA, Walker TM, Bansal A, Setzer WN, Essien EE. Essential oil constituents and biological activities of *Peristrophe bicalyculata* and *Borreria verticillata.* Nat Prod Commun 2010; 5(11): 1815-8.
[http://dx.doi.org/10.1177/1934578X1000501125] [PMID: 21213989]

[88]   Perrone D, Ardito F, Giannatempo G, *et al.* Biological and therapeutic activities, and anticancer properties of curcumin. Exp Ther Med 2015; 10(5): 1615-23.
[http://dx.doi.org/10.3892/etm.2015.2749] [PMID: 26640527]

[89]   Li QS, Li CY, Li ZL, Zhu HL. Genistein and its synthetic analogs as anticancer agents. Anticancer

Agents Med Chem 2012; 12(3): 271-81.
[http://dx.doi.org/10.2174/187152012800228788] [PMID: 22043996]

[90] Bhoopat L, Srichairatanakool S, Kanjanapothi D, Taesotikul T, Thananchai H, Bhoopat T. Hepatoprotective effects of lychee (*Litchi chinensis* Sonn.): a combination of antioxidant and anti-apoptotic activities. J Ethnopharmacol 2011; 136(1): 55-66.
[http://dx.doi.org/10.1016/j.jep.2011.03.061] [PMID: 21540102]

[91] Xiong M, Wang L, Yu HL, *et al.* Ginkgetin exerts growth inhibitory and apoptotic effects on osteosarcoma cells through inhibition of STAT3 and activation of caspase-3/9. Oncol Rep 2016; 35(2): 1034-40.
[http://dx.doi.org/10.3892/or.2015.4427] [PMID: 26573608]

[92] Wang L, Phan DD, Zhang J, *et al.* Anticancer properties of nimbolide and pharmacokinetic considerations to accelerate its development. Oncotarget 2016; 7(28): 44790-802.
[http://dx.doi.org/10.18632/oncotarget.8316] [PMID: 27027349]

[93] Du GJ, Wang CZ, Qi LW, *et al.* The synergistic apoptotic interaction of panaxadiol and epigallocatechin gallate in human colorectal cancer cells. Phytother Res 2013; 27(2): 272-7.
[http://dx.doi.org/10.1002/ptr.4707] [PMID: 22566066]

[94] Liu Y, Yadev VR, Aggarwal BB, Nair MG. Inhibitory effects of black pepper (*Piper nigrum*) extracts and compounds on human tumor cell proliferation, cyclooxygenase enzymes, lipid peroxidation and nuclear transcription factor-kappa-B. Nat Prod Commun 2010; 5(8): 1253-7.
[http://dx.doi.org/10.1177/1934578X1000500822] [PMID: 20839630]

[95] Liu YQ, Tian J, Qian K, *et al.* Recent progress on C-4-modified podophyllotoxin analogs as potent antitumor agents. Med Res Rev 2015; 35(1): 1-62.
[http://dx.doi.org/10.1002/med.21319] [PMID: 24827545]

[96] Pahari P, Saikia UP, Das TP, Damodaran C, Rohr J. Synthesis of Psoralidin derivatives and their anticancer activity: First synthesis of Lespeflorin I^1. Tetrahedron 2016; 72(23): 3324-34.
[http://dx.doi.org/10.1016/j.tet.2016.04.066] [PMID: 27698514]

[97] Al Sinani SS, Eltayeb EA, Coomber BL, Adham SA. Solamargine triggers cellular necrosis selectively in different types of human melanoma cancer cells through extrinsic lysosomal mitochondrial death pathway. Cancer Cell Int 2016; 16: 11.
[http://dx.doi.org/10.1186/s12935-016-0287-4] [PMID: 26889092]

[98] Fakhoury I, Saad W, Bauhadir K, Nygren P, Stock RS, Muhtasib HG. Uptake, delivery and anticancer activity of thymoquinone nanoparticles in breast cancer cells. J Nanopart Res 2016; 18: 210.
[http://dx.doi.org/10.1007/s11051-016-3517-8]

[99] Wozniak L, Skapska S, Marszalek K. Ursolic acid- a pentacyclic triterpenoid with a wide spectrum of pharmacological activities. Molecules 2015; 20(11): 20614-41.
[http://dx.doi.org/10.3390/molecules201119721] [PMID: 26610440]

[100] Lee IC, Choi BY. Withaferin A: a natural anticancer agent with pleiotropic mechanisms of action. Int J Mol Sci 2016; 17(3): 290.
[http://dx.doi.org/10.3390/ijms17030290] [PMID: 26959007]

[101] Vane JR. Inhibition of prostaglandin synthesis as a mechanism of action for aspirin-like drugs. Nat New Biol 1971; 231(25): 232-5.
[http://dx.doi.org/10.1038/newbio231232a0] [PMID: 5284360]

[102] Flower RJ, Moncada S, Vane JR. Analgesic, antipyretics and anti-inflammatory agents: drugs employed in the treatment of gout. The Pharmacological Basis of Therapeutics. New York: Macmillan 1980; p. 682.

[103] Das S, Chatterjee S. Long term toxicity study of ART-400. Indian Ind Med 1995; 16: 117-23.

[104] Dragland S, Senoo H, Wake K, Holte K, Blomhoff R. Several culinary and medicinal herbs are important sources of dietary antioxidants. J Nutr 2003; 133(5): 1286-90.

[http://dx.doi.org/10.1093/jn/133.5.1286] [PMID: 12730411]

[105] Chohan M, Naughton DP, Jones L, Opara EI. An investigation of the relationship between the anti-inflammatory activity, polyphenolic content, and antioxidant activities of cooked and *in vitro* digested culinary herbs. Oxid Med Cell Longev 2012; 2012: 627843.
[http://dx.doi.org/10.1155/2012/627843] [PMID: 22685620]

[106] Wang C, Schuller Levis GB, Lee EB, *et al.* Platycodin D and D3 isolated from the root of *Platycodon grandiflorum* modulate the production of nitric oxide and secretion of TNF-alpha in activated RAW 264.7 cells. Int Immunopharmacol 2004; 4(8): 1039-49.
[http://dx.doi.org/10.1016/j.intimp.2004.04.005] [PMID: 15222978]

[107] Talhouk RS, Karam C, Fostok S, El-Jouni W, Barbour EK. Anti-inflammatory bioactivities in plant extracts. J Med Food 2007; 10(1): 1-10.
[http://dx.doi.org/10.1089/jmf.2005.055] [PMID: 17472460]

[108] Zhang L, Ravipati AS, Koyyalamudi SR, *et al.* Antioxidant and anti-inflammatory activities of selected medicinal plants containing phenolic and flavonoid compounds. J Agric Food Chem 2011; 59(23): 12361-7.
[http://dx.doi.org/10.1021/jf203146e] [PMID: 22023309]

[109] Krishnamoorthy G, Chellappan DR, Joseph J, Ravindhran D, Shabi MM, Uthrapathy S, *et al.* Antioxidant activity of *Nelumbo nucifera* (Gaertn) flowers in isolated perfused rat kidney. Brazilian J Pharmacog 2009; 19(1B): 224-9.
[http://dx.doi.org/10.1590/S0102-695X2009000200008]

[110] Correa WR, Serain AF, Aranha Netto L, *et al.* Anti-inflammatory and antioxidant properties of the extract, tiliroside, and patuletin 3-O-β-D-glucopyranoside from *Pfaffia townsendii* (Amaranthaceae). Evid Based Complement Alternat Med 2018; 20186057579
[http://dx.doi.org/10.1155/2018/6057579] [PMID: 30364020]

[111] Krishnamoorthy G, Dhevi R, Niraimathi KL, Shabi MM, Subashini U, *et al.* Comparative evaluation of *Nelumbo nucifera* Gaertn. flowers and vitamin C in *in-vitro* antioxidant activity. ICFAI University J Life Sci 2009; 3(1): 7-19.

[112] Chemical constituents from *Polygonatum odoratum.* Biochem Syst Ecol 2015; 58: 281-4.
[http://dx.doi.org/10.1016/j.bse.2014.12.019]

[113] Mandal S, Patra A, Samanta A, *et al.* Analysis of phytochemical profile of *Terminalia arjuna* bark extract with antioxidative and antimicrobial properties. Asian Pac J Trop Biomed 2013; 3(12): 960-6.
[http://dx.doi.org/10.1016/S2221-1691(13)60186-0] [PMID: 24093787]

[114] Rastogi S, Iqbal MS, Ohri D. *In vitro* study of anti-inflammatory and antioxidant activity of some medicinal plants and their interrelationship. Asian J Pharm Clinical Res 2018; 11(4): 195-02.
[http://dx.doi.org/10.22159/ajpcr.2018.v11i4.23583]

[115] Chansiw N, Chotinantakul K, Srichairatanakool S. Anti-inflammatory and antioxidant activities of the extracts from leaves and stems of *Polygonumodoratum.* Antiinflamm Antiallergy Agents Med Chem 2019; 18(1): 45-54.
[http://dx.doi.org/10.2174/1871523017666181109144548] [PMID: 30411695]

[116] Shabi MM, Gayathri K, Dhevi R, Subasini U, Victor Rajamanickam G, Dubey GP. *Cardiospermum halicacabum* (Linn): Investigations on anti-inflammatory and analgesic effect. Bulg J Vet Med 2009; 12(3): 171-7.

[117] Shabi MM, Uthrapathy S, Raj CD, *et al.* Analgesic and anti-arthritic effect of *Enicostemma littorale* Blume. Adv Biosci Biotechnol 2014; 5: 1018-24.
[http://dx.doi.org/10.4236/abb.2014.513116]

[118] Subasini U, Rajamanickam GV, Dubey GP, Mohammed Shabi M, Gayathri K. Analgesic and anti-arthritic effect of Corallocarpus epigaeus. Int J Biom 2010; 30(3): 313-7.

[119] Thenmozhi S, Dwivedi S, Chaturvedi M, Dwivedi A, Subasini U. Pharmacognostical,

physicochemical and chromatographic estimation of rhizomes and rhizome oil of *Alpinia speciosa* Roxb. Int J Discov Herb Res 2013; 3(3): 649-51.

[120]   Chao CY, Sung PJ, Wang WH, Kuo YH. Anti-inflammatory effect of *Momordica charantia* in sepsis mice. Molecules 2014; 19(8): 12777-88.
[http://dx.doi.org/10.3390/molecules190812777] [PMID: 25153878]

[121]   Tohma H, GulAin I, Bursal E, Goren AC, Alwasel SH, Koksal E. Antioxidant activity and phenolic compounds of ginger (*Zingiber officinale*Rosc.) determined by HPLC-MS/MS. J Food Meas Charact 2017; 11(2): 556-66.
[http://dx.doi.org/10.1007/s11694-016-9423-z]

[122]   Elosta A, Slevin M, Rahman K, Ahmed N. Aged garlic has more potent antiglycation and antioxidant properties compared to fresh garlic extract *in vitro.* Sci Rep 2017; 7: 39613.
[http://dx.doi.org/10.1038/srep39613] [PMID: 28051097]

[123]   Mathur A, Verma SK. Reena Purohit R, Singh SK, Mathur D, Prasad GBKS, Dua VK. Pharmacological investigation of *Bacopa monnieri* on the basis of antioxidant, antimicrobial and anti-inflammatory properties. J Chem Pharm Res 2010; 2(6): 191-8.

[124]   Kaurinovic B, Popovic M, Vlaisavljevic S, Trivic S. Antioxidant capacity of *Ocimum basilicum* L. and *Origanum vulgare* L. extracts. Molecules 2011; 16(9): 7401-14.
[http://dx.doi.org/10.3390/molecules16097401] [PMID: 21878860]

[125]   Maizura M, Aminah A, Wan Aida WM. Total phenolic content and antioxidant activity of kesum (*Polygonum minus*), ginger (*Zingiber officinale*) and turmeric (*Curcuma longa*) extract. Int Food Res J 2011; 18(2): 322-34.

[126]   Gacche RN, Dhole NA. Antioxidant and anti-inflammatory potential of selected medicines plants prescribed in Indian traditional system of medicine. Pharma Biol J 2008; 44(5): 389-95.
[http://dx.doi.org/10.1080/13880200600751691]

[127]   Raymond N, Nono RN. Antioxidant anti-inflammatory activities of extract from roots of *Dissotis thollonii*cogn. S Afr J Bot 2014; 93: 1-2.

[128]   Poyton RO, Ball KA, Castello PR. Mitochondrial generation of free radicals and hypoxic signaling. Trends Endocrinol Metab 2009; 20(7): 332-40.
[http://dx.doi.org/10.1016/j.tem.2009.04.001] [PMID: 19733481]

[129]   Knopp RH. Risk factors for coronary artery disease in women. Am J Cardiol 2002; 89 (12A): 28E-34E.
[http://dx.doi.org/10.1016/S0002-9149(02)02409-8] [PMID: 12084401]

[130]   Huang WC, Lin TW, Chiou KR, *et al.* The effect of intensified low-density lipoprotein cholesterol reduction on recurrent myocardial infarction and cardiovascular mortality. Acta Cardiol Sin 2013; 29(5): 404-12.
[PMID: 27122737]

[131]   Stone NJ, Robinson JG, Lichtenstein AH, *et al.* ACC/AHA guideline on the treatment of blood cholesterol to reduce atherosclerotic cardiovascular risk in adults: a report of the American College of Cardiology/American Heart Association Task Force on Practice Guidelines Circulation 129(25 Suppl 2)2014; S1-S45..

[132]   Khan A, Maki KC, Ito MK, *et al.* Statin associated muscle symptoms: characteristics of patients and recommendations by providers. J Clin Lipidol 2015; 9(3): 460.
[http://dx.doi.org/10.1016/j.jacl.2015.03.080]

[133]   Bitzur R, Cohen H, Kamari Y, Harats D. Intolerance to statins: mechanisms and management. Diabetes Care 2013; 36 (Suppl. 2): S325-30.
[http://dx.doi.org/10.2337/dcS13-2038] [PMID: 23882066]

[134]   Bang CN, Okin PM. Statin treatment, new-onset diabetes, and other adverse effects: a systematic review. Curr Cardiol Rep 2014; 16(3): 461.

[http://dx.doi.org/10.1007/s11886-013-0461-4] [PMID: 24464306]

[135]   Ojha S, Bhatia J, Arora S, Golechha M, Kumari S, Arya DS. Cardioprotective effects of *Commiphora mukul* against isoprenaline-induced cardiotoxicity: a biochemical and histopathological evaluation. J Environ Biol 2011; 32(6): 731-8.
[PMID: 22471209]

[136]   Subramaniam S, Ramachandran S, Uthrapathi S, Gnamanickam VR, Dubey GP. Anti-hyperlipidemic and antioxidant potential of different fractions of *Terminalia arjuna* Roxb. bark against PX- 407 induced hyperlipidemia. Indian J Exp Biol 2011; 49(4): 282-8.
[PMID: 21614892]

[137]   Subasini U, Shabi MM, Gayathri K, *et al.* Phytochemical evaluation with hypoglycaemic and antioxidant activity of *Tribulus terrestris* Linn. Intern J Biomed 2009; 29(2): 121-7.

[138]   Nandave M, Ojha SK, Joshi S, Kumari S, Arya DS. Cardioprotective effect of *Bacopa monneira* against isoproterenol-induced myocardial necrosis in rats. Int J Pharmacol 2007; 3(5): 385-92.
[http://dx.doi.org/10.3923/ijp.2007.385.392]

[139]   Suchal K, Bhatia J, Malik S, *et al.* Sea buckthorn pulp oil protects against myocardial ischemia-reperfusion injury in rats through activation of Akt/Enos. Front Pharmacol 2016; 7(7): 155.
[http://dx.doi.org/10.3389/fphar.2016.00155] [PMID: 27445803]

[140]   Lukmanul H, Girija A, Boopathy R. Antioxidant property of selected Ocimum species their secondary metabolite content. J Med Plants Res 2008; 2(9): 250-7.

[141]   Temitope AG, Sheriff O, Taofik A, Fatimah AZ. Cardioprotective properties of *Momordica charantia* in albino rats. Afr J Sci Res 2013; 11(1): 600-10.

[142]   Isensee H, Rietz B, Jacob R. Cardioprotective actions of garlic (*Allium sativum*). Arzneimittelforschung 1993; 43(2): 94-8.
[PMID: 8457243]

[143]   Chan JY, Yuen AC, Chan RY, Chan SW. A review of the cardiovascular benefits and antioxidant properties of Allicin Phyto other Res. 2013; 27: pp. 637- 646.

[144]   Kataria R. pharmacological activities on *Glycyrrhiza glabra* -a review. Asian J Pharm Clin Res 2013; 6(1): 5-7.

[145]   Sun CM, Syu WJ, Don MJ, Lu JJ, Lee GH. Cytotoxic sesquiterpene lactones from the root of Saussurea lappa. J Nat Prod 2003; 66(9): 1175-80.
[http://dx.doi.org/10.1021/np030147e] [PMID: 14510592]

[146]   Shafiq H, Ahmad A, Masud T, Kaleem M. Cardio-protective and anti-cancer therapeutic potential of *Nigella sativa.* Iran J Basic Med Sci 2014; 17(12): 967-79.
[PMID: 25859300]

[147]   Narayanaswamy N, Balakrishnan KP. Evaluation of some medicinal plants for their antioxidant properties. Int J Pharm Tech Res 2011; 3(1): 381-5.

[148]   Nagaraju D, Vidhyadhara S. Evaluation of cardioprotective activity of ethanolic extract of dried leaves of *Cinnamomum tamala* in rats. Int J Biol Adv Res 2016; 7(4): 181-6.
[http://dx.doi.org/10.7439/ijbar.v7i4.3211]

[149]   Upagnalwar A, Balarama R. Cardioprotective effects of *Lagenaria siceraria* fruit juice on isoproterenol induced myocardial infraction in Wistar rats. A biochemical and Histo architecture study. J Young Pharmacists 2011; 3(4): 297-303.
[http://dx.doi.org/10.4103/0975-1483.90241]

[150]   Rifat-uz-Zaman, Study of cardioprotective activity of *Raphanus sativus* in rabbits. Pak J Biol Sci 2004; 843-7 :(5)7. [http://dx.doi.org/10.3923/pjbs.2004.843.847]

[151]   Rao PR, Kumar VK, Viswanath RK, Subbaraju GV. Cardioprotective activity of alcoholic extract of *Tinospora cordifolia* in ischemia-reperfusion induced myocardial infarction in rats. Biol Pharm Bull

2005; 28(12): 2319-22.
[http://dx.doi.org/10.1248/bpb.28.2319] [PMID: 16327173]

[152] Prabhu S, Jainu M, Sabitha KE, Devi CS. Cardioprotective effect of mangiferin on isoproterenol induced myocardial infarction in rats. Indian J Exp Biol 2006; 44(3): 209-15.
[PMID: 16538859]

[153] Kinattingala N, Mahalakshmia AM, Manjula SN. Cardioprotective effect of *Tamarindus indica* Linn against isoproterenol induced myocardial infraction in rats. Int J Pharm 2016; 8(5): 254-60.

[154] Ziberna L, Lunder M. Mozos, Vanzo A, Drensek G. Cardioprotective effects of bilberry extract on is chemia reperfusion induced injury in isolated rat heart. BMC Pharmacol 2009; 9(2): A55.
[http://dx.doi.org/10.1186/1471-2210-9-S2-A55]

[155] Kaur S, Mondal P. Study of total phenolic and flavonoid content, antioxidant activity and antimicrobial properties of medicinal plants. J Microbiol Exp 2014; 1(1): 1-6.
[http://dx.doi.org/10.15406/jmen.2014.01.00005]

[156] Dhiman A, La R, Bhan M, Dhiman B, Hooda A. Plebeian assessment of anti-microbial and *in vitro* antioxidant zest of *Datura fastuosa* L. seeds. J Pharma Sci Innov 2012; 1(4): 49-53.

[157] Nammi S, Koka S, Chinnala KM, Boini KM. Obesity: an overview on its current perspectives and treatment options. Nutr J 2004; 3: 3.
[http://dx.doi.org/10.1186/1475-2891-3-3] [PMID: 15084221]

[158] Azain MJ. Role of fatty acids in adipocyte growth and development. J Anim Sci 2004; 82(3): 916-24.
[http://dx.doi.org/10.2527/2004.823916x] [PMID: 15032450]

[159] Bray GA, Tartaglia LA. Medicinal strategies in the treatment of obesity. Nature 2000; 404(6778): 672-7.
[http://dx.doi.org/10.1038/35007544] [PMID: 10766254]

[160] (World Health Organization), Obesity: preventing and managing the global epidemic Report of a WHO Consultation on Obesity. Geneva: WHO 1998.

[161] National Family Health Survey. International Institute for Population Sciences (IIPS) and ORC Macro, 1998-99, Mumbai: IIPS, NFHS-2. 2000.

[162] Flum DR, Salem L, Elrod JA, Dellinger EP, Cheadle A, Chan L. Early mortality among Medicare beneficiaries undergoing bariatric surgical procedures. JAMA 2005; 294(15): 1903-8.
[http://dx.doi.org/10.1001/jama.294.15.1903] [PMID: 16234496]

[163] Van Gaal LF, Rissanen AM, Scheen AJ, Ziegler O, RAssner S. Effects of the cannabinoid-1 receptor blocker rimonabant on weight reduction and cardiovascular risk factors in overweight patients: 1-year experience from the RIO-Europe study. Lancet 2005; 365(9468): 1389-97.
[http://dx.doi.org/10.1016/S0140-6736(05)66374-X] [PMID: 15836887]

[164] Surh YJ. Anti-tumor promoting potential of selected spice ingredients with antioxidative and anti-inflammatory activities: a short review. Food Chem Toxicol 2002; 40(8): 1091-7.
[http://dx.doi.org/10.1016/S0278-6915(02)00037-6] [PMID: 12067569]

[165] Hasani-Ranjbar S, Larijani B, Abdollahi M. A systematic review of Iranian medicinal plants useful in diabetes mellitus. Arch Med Sci 2008; 4: 285-92.

[166] Gholamhoseinian A, Shahouzehi B, Sharififar F. Inhibitory effect of some plant extract on pancreatic lipase. Int J Pharmacol 2010; 6: 18-24.
[http://dx.doi.org/10.3923/ijp.2010.18.24]

[167] Han LK, Takaku T, Li J, Kimura Y, Okuda H. Anti-obesity action of oolong tea. Int J Obes Relat Metab Disord 1999; 23(1): 98-105.
[http://dx.doi.org/10.1038/sj.ijo.0800766] [PMID: 10094584]

[168] Ninomiya K, Matsuda H, Shimoda H, *et al.* Carnosic acid, a new class of lipid absorption inhibitor from sage. Bioorg Med Chem Lett 2004; 14(8): 1943-6.

[http://dx.doi.org/10.1016/j.bmcl.2004.01.091] [PMID: 15050633]

[169] Yun JW. Possible anti-obesity therapeutics from nature--a review. Phytochemistry 2010; 71(14-15): 1625-41.
[http://dx.doi.org/10.1016/j.phytochem.2010.07.011] [PMID: 20732701]

SUBJECT INDEX

Javed Ahmad and Javed Ahamad (Eds.)

www.ingramcontent.com/pod-product-compliance
Lightning Source LLC
Chambersburg PA
CBHW050832220326
41598CB00006B/354